FOOD POLITICS

WHAT EVERYONE NEEDS TO KNOW®

FOOD POLITICS

WHAT EVERYONE NEEDS TO KNOW®

Third Edition

ROBERT PAARLBERG

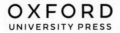

OXFORD
UNIVERSITY PRESS

Oxford University Press is a department of the University of Oxford. It furthers the University's objective of excellence in research, scholarship, and education by publishing worldwide. Oxford is a registered trade mark of Oxford University Press in the UK and certain other countries.

"What Everyone Needs to Know" is a registered trademark of Oxford University Press.

Published in the United States of America by Oxford University Press 198 Madison Avenue, New York, NY 10016, United States of America.

© Oxford University Press 2023

CIP data is on file at the Library of Congress

ISBN 978–0–19–774377–5 (pbk.)
ISBN 978–0–19–774376–8 (hbk.)

DOI: 10.1093/wentk/9780197743768.001.0001

Paperback printed by Sheridan Books, Inc., United States of America
Hardback printed by Bridgeport National Bindery, Inc., United States of America

CONTENTS

PREFACE TO THE THIRD EDITION OF FOOD POLITICS

I have enjoyed preparing this third edition of *Food Politics: What Everyone Needs to Know*, because it has reminded me of important changes seen in food and farm politics around the world since the second edition was published in 2013. Since that time, three unexpected events temporarily disrupted the policy environment. First was President Trump's trade war with China, which interrupted America's exports of soybeans and pork when China retaliated. Second was the COVID-19 pandemic beginning in 2020, which put supply chains under stress and locked down food service in large parts of the world. Third was the 2022 war in Ukraine, which interrupted wheat and fertilizer exports, and which at this writing is still underway.

Political and policy change was also driven by four more powerful and durable factors: the continued rise of China, scientific discoveries (including a new genetic improvement method for crops and animals named CRISPR), innovations from food entrepreneurs (such as plant-based and cell-grown imitation meats), and of course climate change. I agreed with my editor at Oxford that such developments together, in addition to many smaller changes plus the simple passage of time, had altered the food politics landscape enough to justify a new edition of the book.

Since the previous edition of *Food Politics*, my own professional involvement in food and farming has continued and deepened, both within the university world and beyond. As the chair of an independent steering committee for a Consultative Group on International Agricultural Research program on Agriculture for Nutrition and Health (A4NH), I have been in a position to review research projects in nutrition as well as farming, making visits to field sites in Nigeria, Ethiopia, Bangladesh, and Vietnam. I also continued to serve as a consultant to the International Food Policy Research Institute (IFPRI), conducting a series of impact assessments for that organization, and for four years I worked as a co-investigator on a R01 grant from the National Institutes of Health, on policy strategies to improve diets and reduce cardiovascular disease in the United States. This project led to the publication of academic journal articles on sugar-sweetened beverage taxes and on efforts to strengthen health impacts in the SNAP (food stamp) program. Then in 2021, I joined a Task Force on Food and Nutrition Security at the Bipartisan Policy Center in Washington, DC, to prepare policy briefs for the 2023 farm bill.

Since the second edition of *Food Politics*, I have also written two additional books. One was published in 2015 by Oxford University Press, titled *The United States of Excess*. This book explained why America has been a global outlier in its excessive consumption of both food and fossil fuel. The other book, published in 2021 by Knopf, was written for a popular audience and is titled *Resetting the Table: Straight Talk About the Food We Grow and Eat*. In 2022, this book won a Nautilus Book Award in the category of sustainability.

As in earlier editions, I should share with curious readers some information about my family background, because political perspectives are invariably shaped by personal experiences. My father was raised on a farm in Indiana, became a professor of agricultural economics and then a senior government official, and passed along to me his interests in public policy and international travel, plus an agrarian heritage I am proud to celebrate. My concern for rural poverty and undernutrition dates from an early visit I made to India and Nepal, where my brother was serving as a Peace Corps volunteer. I returned later to study the evolution of food and farming policies in South Asia, and eventually worked in more than a dozen countries in Africa as well, where my active research efforts remain ongoing. In this book I try to keep my own personal perspectives in their proper place, but I cannot pretend they are absent.

I take pride in my independence; in my long career as a university-based academic, I have never been funded or employed by any private company. My research has sometimes been funded by private foundations, and sometimes by governmental or intergovernmental agencies, but most often I turned for research support to the generosity of my longtime employer, Wellesley College. I want to take another opportunity here to thank this wonderful institution. As for my political leanings, I have always been a registered Democrat, yet my views on food and farming do not fall neatly into partisan categories. The sections of this book that address food trade and science-based farming are likely to irritate some of my fellow Democrats, and please the political Right, but the sections that address food companies, development assistance, climate change, and animal welfare are likely to do the opposite.

In modern societies where few people still work the land as full-time farmers, and where markets offer an ever wider range of choices about what to eat, how to eat, and how much to eat, the politics of food has come to extend far beyond material questions of who gets what, or even Left versus Right. Nor is there a unified perspective among academic specialists. Biologists and economists are routinely challenged on such matters by philosophers, ecologists, and sociologists. Originally trained as a political scientist, I try to remain open to multiple perspectives.

I share with food activists considerable dissatisfaction with today's world of food and farming. Too much of our food is unhealthy, too much of our farming is still unsustainable, too many farm workers are underpaid, and too many of our rural societies remain unjust. Our world of 8 billion food consumers is still not being adequately or properly fed. I may be less scolding toward our world food system than some, and also less pessimistic about the future, but I see the value of pessimism in motivating political leaders to act. I offer this updated and revised edition of *Food Politics: What Everyone Needs to Know* as a fresh starting point for problem solvers of every stripe, in hopes it will inform motivated actions both now and in the years ahead.

FOOD POLITICS

WHAT EVERYONE NEEDS TO KNOW®

1

AN OVERVIEW OF
FOOD POLITICS

What is food politics?

Since biblical times, the policies of governments have shaped food and farming. The book of Genesis (47:24) records that in Egypt the pharaoh took 20 percent of all food production from his farmers as a tax. Some governments in modern-day Africa burden farmers nearly as much, by maintaining overvalued exchange rates that favor urban food consumers over rural food producers, and by failing to invest in rural infrastructure like roads, power, or irrigation. Conversely, governments in wealthy industrial countries provide direct and indirect subsidies to farmers, typically at the expense of both taxpayers and consumers. Understanding the political dynamics behind such differences between agricultural versus post-agricultural societies is one of the goals of this book.

The food and farming sectors of all states, ancient and modern, are the site of considerable political activity. Rural food producers and urban food consumers have divergent short-term interests, so they naturally compete for control of the far-reaching powers of the state (e.g., collecting taxes, providing subsidies, managing exchange rates, regulating markets), hoping to pursue a self-serving advantage. We describe such struggles over how the risks and gains from state action will be allocated within the food and farming sector as "food politics." The distinctive feature of food politics is not just social disagreement over food, but political competition to shape the actions of government. If you and I have a personal difference over the wisdom of eating junk food, that by itself is not food politics, but if you and your allies organize to advocate new government regulations on junk food (e.g., restricting what can be served in public school cafeterias), the disagreement becomes food politics.

Is food politics driven by material interests or by social values?

Food politics is driven by both. In poor countries where large numbers of citizens still work in the farming sector and often find it difficult between harvests to afford enough food, material interests will tend to dominate. In these societies, food and farming are still a large part of material welfare for all. In wealthy post-agricultural societies, however, farmers are few in number, and most consumers can easily afford an adequate diet. In these societies, material conflicts around food and farming will persist, but social values—such as values regarding the natural environment, or toward animal welfare, or toward the preservation of traditional communities—will begin to play a larger role.

Country by country, food politics is often similar to other kinds of politics. In democratic societies, it revolves around the actions of elected government officials who confront pressures from organized non-governmental groups in society. In authoritarian or one-party states, it emerges from official rulings issued by political elites who are less accountable to society. Yet food politics does exhibit a consistent pattern across all countries, linked to a larger process of industrial and post-industrial development. Industrialization brings rapid productivity growth to both farming and manufacturing, but it also brings a rapid reduction in farm employment, as fewer people are needed to produce food. In the United States, the share of farmers in the workforce fell from 50 percent in 1870 to only 3 percent by 1990, and to just 1 percent today. Meanwhile, the growth of urban population and income boosts the demand for food and brings a rapid expansion of food-processing companies, private food transport and distribution systems, supermarkets, and food service restaurants. At every step in this process, politically motivated groups of farmers and non-farmers, private companies, and non-governmental organizations will struggle to shape government policy in a manner consistent with their preferences.

As the farming sector begins to lose its numerical strength, farmers will organize to take political action and seek government support. In the United States, Europe, and Japan during the peak decades of industrialization in the mid-20th century, farmer organizations demanded escalating subsidies from the state and those subsidies were provided. By the 1980s, farmers in Japan were getting $23 billion worth of farm program benefits from their government, farmers in the United States were getting $26 billion, and farmers in the European Community (a predecessor to the European Union) were getting $33 billion.

When these wealthy societies later moved into a post-industrial stage of development, the subsidy policies originally set in place to benefit struggling farmers lost much of their original rationale, because most who remained on farms were no longer struggling. In the United States, the average income for farm families in 2019 was 26 percent above the average for all households. Under these new circumstances, political advocacy around food production shifted away from farm income support and toward health concerns such as pesticide residues, environmental concerns such as chemical use or greenhouse gas emissions, and "food movement" concerns such as animal welfare or rebuilding local food systems.

Political struggles over food and farm policy within these democratic societies are divisive and polarizing because the opposing positions often rest on conflicting social values, making compromise difficult. Debates over conventional versus organic farming, or over industrial versus small-scale livestock production, or over supermarkets versus farmers' markets, provide little space for policy agreement. Yet the policies that emerge in democratic states are typically more successful than those within authoritarian or one-party systems. In authoritarian states, where individuals and groups in society lack an institutionalized political voice, serious food policy errors are frequently made. In fact, serious famines have only taken place in nondemocratic societies. The worst famine ever recorded took place in China in 1959–1961, during the so-called Great Leap Forward, when radical policy decisions made by the unchallenged ruler Mao Zedong caused an estimated 30 million people to die of hunger. The world's most recent famines have also taken place in nondemocratic states: in North Korea after 1996, in southern Somalia in 2011, and in South Sudan in 2017.

Is food politics a global or a local phenomenon?

One widely quoted legislative leader in the United States, Representative Tip O'Neill from Massachusetts, famously said, "All politics is local." This holds true for much of food politics. Analysts like to talk about the "world food system," but to a large extent the world's people continue to rely on many separate national or even local food systems. Wheat is the most heavily traded food commodity, yet 75 percent of the world's wheat consumption is satisfied from domestic supplies. For rice, only 10 percent of global consumption is supplied by imports. In the poorest agricultural countries, a great deal of the food available is still consumed within the same community that produced it, or even by the same individual who produced it. When understanding the food politics of such countries, it will usually be local weather, local markets, local social conditions, and the actions of local leaders that will matter most.

The heaviest users of international food markets are today's rich (overfed) countries, not poor underfed countries, and much of what the rich import is feed for animals, not food for direct human consumption. For example, the world's biggest corn buyer is China, which imported $7.6 billion worth of corn in 2021, almost all for animal feed. China is also the world's biggest importer of soybeans, again mostly for animal feed. For food staple crops like rice, China has traditionally limited its imports in the name of food "self-sufficiency." Japan and South Korea have done the same. Many large countries in Asia, including India and Pakistan, have sought to avoid rice imports entirely. Such policies frustrate food-exporting countries including the United States, and they violate the pro-trade advice of international bodies such as the World Trade Organization (WTO), but separate national governments give international food markets only so much room to operate.

In addition to remaining significantly compartmentalized, the world's food and farming systems produce nutrition outcomes that diverge dramatically country by country, and also person by person within countries. When it comes to food and agriculture, the world is far from flat. The wealthy regions of Europe, North America, and East Asia are agriculturally productive and well fed (increasingly, they are overfed), while the less wealthy regions of South Asia and tropical Africa are still home to hundreds of millions of farmers who are not yet highly productive and large numbers of people who are not adequately nourished. In Sub-Saharan Africa today, about 60 percent of all citizens are smallholder farmers or herdsmen living in the countryside, and one out of three is chronically undernourished. In South Asia, roughly 60 percent of the population is engaged in agriculture, and in India in 2022 the average income of farm households was less than $6 a day. Many control no land of their own and must work as hired laborers. The material needs of poor farmers in these regions remain unmet in part because their national governments have underinvested in rural roads, water, power, schools, and clinics. The rural poor have scant political power (many are women with little schooling, unable to read or write), so they are all too easy for governments to ignore.

In some settings, the politics of food and farming is addressed within a global frame of reference. For example, agricultural trade restrictions have been the subject of periodic global negotiations at the WTO, where nearly all nations have membership, and global food assistance needs are addressed by the UN World Food Programme (WFP), another universal body. Yet national and local food and farming systems remain significantly separate and divided, thanks to geographic distance, weak transport infrastructures, divergent cultural and dietary traditions, and large gaps in purchasing power. These diverse and largely separate food systems are shaped by the policies of separate national governments, many of which have different capabilities, distinct characteristics, and divergent priorities. As a result, most policy success or failure in food and farming takes place nationally or locally, rather than globally. Thinking globally is good advice when working on problems such as climate change, pandemics, telecommunications policy, or international finance, but when considering the politics of food and agriculture, it is often more useful to think nationally, and sometimes even locally.

Who are the most important actors in food politics?

Food politics takes place both inside and outside of government, among multiple organizations with divergent preferences that compete with each other for influence. Organizations representing consumers will usually want food prices to be low, while advocates for farmers usually want high crop prices (except livestock producers, who will want cheap grain for feeding to animals). In addition, farmers' organizations will typically campaign against tight environmental regulations in their sector, supported by the industries that supply them with inputs such as fertilizer and pesticides. Environmental organizations will campaign for tighter regulations. Groups claiming to speak for consumers will line up against food and beverage companies when the issue is food safety or nutrition labeling requirements. Growers that hire seasonal farm workers will want lenient visa requirements for labor migrants, while labor unions promoting higher wages will prefer the opposite.

In countries with democratic political systems, each of these groups will cultivate its own special friends and supporters inside government, especially within elected legislatures. In the United States, the organizations seeking assistance for commercial farmers are known as "farm lobbies," and they make generous campaign contributions to members of the agricultural committees of Congress, ensuring that once every five years those members will support new legislation (a new "farm bill") renewing the generous entitlement programs that provide income subsidies to farmers. To guarantee a majority vote, food purchase subsidies that benefit low-income households will be included in the bill, ensuring support from members representing urban districts. This is a standard legislative tactic known as a "committee-based logroll." Taxpayers will usually be the biggest losers when the logs start to roll.

Has the politics of food and agriculture recently been changing?

In today's advanced industrial and post-industrial societies, especially in Europe and North America, the politics of food and agriculture has recently undergone significant change. There was a time when food consumers in these societies wanted just four things: foods that were safe, plentiful in variety, more convenient to purchase and prepare, and lower in cost. Now consumers in these countries routinely demand other things as well, such as foods grown without synthetic chemicals (organic), foods that can satisfy new dietary preferences (vegan, gluten-free, ketogenic, etc.), foods grown with a smaller carbon footprint, foods that are locally grown on small farms, and foods produced with less harm to farm animals. Emerging tastes of this kind among increasingly affluent and aware consumers have not driven low-cost convenience foods off the market by any means, but niche markets are now growing rapidly for foods that are local, organic, "climate smart," or "humanely produced." These alternatives frequently dominate social debate, and in the United States, advocates for these alternative approaches see themselves as part of a new social movement—a "food movement"—attempting to exercise hard political power, not just soft cultural influence. In 2013, *New York Times* food columnist Mark Bittman likened today's emergence of such a movement to other important historic struggles for change, such as the battle to abolish slavery and the long struggle to extend voting rights to women.

Within the political arena, however, lobbyists working on behalf of conventional food industries and large commercial farmers have continued to retain the upper hand. Much to the frustration of nutrition activists, food writers, advocates for farm animal welfare, and proponents of organic or local farms, most food and farming sectors continue to move toward greater consolidation, greater automation, more industrialization, and more rather than less globalization. Yet in cultural terms, new battle lines have been drawn, and conventional food and farming industries know they are under attack. Political leaders, caught in the middle, can find it impossible to satisfy both camps.

These new political battles over food and farming are also being projected outward, beyond today's post-industrial societies into middle-income and transitional societies, and even into poor countries that are still largely agrarian in character. Through trade and foreign assistance policies; foreign investment actions by multinational food companies, supermarkets, and restaurant chains; and the countervailing advocacy by non-governmental civil society organizations (NGOs) critical of conventional food and agriculture, rich post-industrial societies have been exporting their new debates over food and farming to the rest of the world. In commercial terms, the food systems of the world are far from fully integrated, yet the terms of modern debate over food and farm policy have been globalized to a surprising degree.

2

FOOD PRODUCTION AND POPULATION GROWTH

Who was Thomas Malthus, and why did he see hunger as inevitable?

Thomas Robert Malthus was an English economist who authored in 1798 a highly influential treatise, *An Essay on the Principle of Population*. In this essay, Malthus argued that food production could never stay ahead of population growth because it would be constrained by the farmland available, an asset that can expand only slowly, while human population tends to grow exponentially. Malthus concluded, "The power of population is so superior to the power of the earth to produce subsistence for man, that premature death must in some shape or other visit the human race." Malthus meant premature death from war, plague, illness, or widespread famine.

Predicting a future of war, plague, and famine was credible enough in 1798, since these had all been recurring tragedies throughout history until then. Yet it was entirely new to predict—as Malthus did—that these tragedies were sure to worsen in the future due to the inability of agriculture to keep pace with human fertility.

Was Malthus right? In 1798, when he wrote his treatise, the earth had a population only one-tenth as large as today, so numbers of people have increased exponentially, just as Malthus foresaw. The frequency of premature death from hunger and famine has not increased, however. The much larger numbers of people living today typically experience many fewer early deaths, and they tend to be far better fed than in Malthus's time. In England, where Malthus wrote, life expectancy at birth has doubled over the past 200 years, from 40 years then to about 80 years now. So on his own terms, Malthus seems spectacularly wrong.

Yet what about the next 200 years? The earth's population is still increasing, and determined Malthusians insist his prediction might yet come true. Dramatic food production gains since 1798 allowed the human population to grow from 800 million up to 8 billion without any increased frequency of premature death, but the activities of this much larger global population might now do such damage to the environment—including the climate—as to undercut future food production. If environmental damage speeds up while the human population continues to increase (up to more than 10 billion by 2100 according to one UN projection), perhaps a limit will be reached and a Malthusian tragedy will be the result.

Most suspect this will not happen. As agricultural science has advanced, the amount of land and water needed to produce each added bushel of food has declined sharply, reducing harm to the natural environment. For example, the United States today is producing five times as much corn as it did in 1940, on 20 percent *less* land. One study done at Rockefeller University in 2012 concluded that agricultural innovations worldwide had already brought the expansion of global agricultural cropland to a halt, even though both population and food consumption per capita were continuing to rise. This study projected that over the coming 50 years, 360 million acres of land would actually be released from farming globally, an area two and a half times the size of France. If so, this would reverse the Malthusian land constraint on food production.

Was Malthus ever influential?

Malthus may have been consistently wrong for the first two centuries after he made his prediction, but this did not prevent him from being highly influential, particularly among political elites in England in the 19th century. His influence had damaging consequences, particularly in England's colonial territories. Malthus himself was at one point employed as a professor at the British East India Company training college, and his fatalistic views regarding hunger came to influence England's official policies under the Raj, resulting in an indifferent attitude toward the "inevitable" famines that ravaged India during colonial rule. Malthusian thinking also worsened the horrible tragedy of the 1845–1849 Irish famine, caused by a potato blight that decimated Ireland's principal food crop. England controlled Ireland at the time, and political elites in London did little at first to provide relief, in part because they judged the famine to be an inevitable Malthusian consequence of Irish parents producing too many children. It was only because England's political elites embraced Malthusian fatalism that this tragic vision came true.

Fortunately, Malthusian predictions were failing elsewhere at this time because the assumption that food production would remain tightly constrained by the limited land area on earth was shown to be deeply flawed. Land constraints were progressively lifted beginning in the 19th century, thanks to the application of modern science to farming. A cascade of new farming technologies emerged over the two centuries after Malthus wrote his *Essay*—especially synthetic nitrogen fertilizer and improved seed varieties—that allowed crop production on existing farmland to skyrocket. An acre of land today can produce more than 10 times as much food as it could when Malthus wrote in 1798.

These science-based crop-yield gains were particularly dramatic during the second half of the 20th century. In the United States, average corn yields increased from 34 bushels an acre in the 1940s to 121 bushels per acre by the 1990s and then to 147 bushels per acre by 2011. Yields of corn well above 200 bushels an acre are now common among farmers using the best new seeds and the most sophisticated practices. Farm productivity increased so rapidly in the 20th century that the price of food declined (the "real" price, discounting for inflation), even though population and food demand were both steeply on the rise. The real price of farm commodities fell by more than 50 percent in the United States between 1900 and 2000, despite unprecedented consumption increases driven by high income growth as well as population growth.

Malthus also misjudged long-term trends in human fertility. By assuming birthrates would remain continuously high, he failed to anticipate the reduction in family size that takes place when societies become wealthier and more urbanized. In urban societies, the value of having large families for unskilled farm labor declines while payoffs increase from concentrating education investments on fewer children, so family size shrinks. Fertility also tends to fall when more children begin surviving infancy thanks to improved medical practices, and once education and employment opportunities are extended to young women as well as young men. This always leads to later marriage and hence to fewer years of active childbearing per woman. Because of all these factors in combination, fertility has dropped sharply in all modern industrial societies, and population growth has slowed as a consequence.

In most European countries today, population is actually shrinking—and not due to premature deaths from war, plague, or famine. Fertility (births per woman of child-bearing age) in all European countries is now below the level required for full replacement of the population in the long run (around 2.1 children per woman), and in the majority of cases fertility has been below this replacement level for several decades. Rapidly declining fertility is also now notable in India, Indonesia, Brazil, and Mexico. As a result, for the first time ever there are more people on the planet today over 65 than under 5.

These declines in fertility have reduced the United Nations (UN) projection of the earth's peak population from 12 billion down to just 10 billion. Malthus has thus been doubly wrong so far. He expected that fertility would remain high, in the face of lagging food production, but instead we see fertility dropping steeply, even as food production continues a rapid global increase. Africa remains something of an exception, because food production there is not rapidly increasing even as population growth remains strong. But the good news in Africa is that much of today's population growth reflects a fortunate increase in rates of child survival. African birth rates per woman are actually falling sharply, but child death rates are falling even more.

Are Malthusians still influential?

In the 20th century, Malthusian anxieties peaked in the 1960s and 1970s, a time of high population growth in Asia, particularly in India and Bangladesh. In 1967, brothers William and Paul Paddock, an agronomist and a former Department of State official respectively, wrote a best-seller titled *Famine 1975!*, which projected that India would never be able to feed its growing population. The Paddocks even warned it would be a mistake to give food aid to India because that would keep people alive just long enough to have still more children, leading to even more starvation in the future. Fortunately, this advice was not taken. The US government delivered unprecedented quantities of food aid to India in the 1960s to offset poor harvests, and outsiders also helped India invest in a significant upgrade of its own farming operations—an upgrade that came to be known as the "green revolution." Improved seeds and fertilizers allowed India's farmers to boost their production of wheat and rice dramatically, and by 1975, India was able to end food aid deliveries completely, without a famine.

Paul R. Ehrlich, an American entomologist who originally specialized in butterflies, made a parallel Malthusian argument in a 1968 best-seller titled *The Population Bomb*. Ehrlich predicted that hundreds of millions would die in the 1970s due to excessive population growth. His began his book with a memorable pronouncement: "The battle to feed all of humanity is over." Ehrlich even projected that by 1980, residents in the United States would have a life expectancy of only 42 years. Surprisingly, this book continues to be cited, a stubborn persistence of Malthusian fatalism in the face of contrary evidence.

Can we feed a growing population without doing irreversible damage to the environment?

Modern-day Malthusians often add both a dietary and an environmental component to their arguments. Regarding diet, they note that each individual today is more likely to consume larger quantities of animal products—meat, milk, and eggs—increasing the need for agricultural land to produce animal feed. Even before climate change arose as their top concern, environmentalists feared that pushing food production to keep pace with population would result in too many dry lands or forest lands being cleared for farming, and too much groundwater or surface water being used for farm irrigation. Biodiversity and wildlife habitat would be lost. Food production might continue increasing in the short run, but eventually a combination of falling water tables caused by over-pumping, plus desertification caused by the plowing and grazing of dry lands, could push production gains into reverse. This would bring an even more devastating Malthusian collapse, because by then the human population would be even larger. Under this scenario, the most frightening thought is that we may have already exceeded the earth's capacity for *sustainable* food production without realizing it.

Eco-Malthusian "overshoot and collapse" projections of this kind have been in circulation at least since a 1972 report from an organization called the Club of Rome, titled *Limits to Growth*.

Jared Diamond's 2005 best-selling book titled *Collapse: How Societies Choose to Fail or Succeed* also popularized the overshoot idea. Diamond's account of the disastrous fate of early peoples on Easter Island, Greenland, and the Maya in Central America was offered to drive home the importance of staying within eco-Malthusian limits. Diamond's weakness was that he could only document overshoot and collapse vulnerabilities among pre-scientific societies lacking the innovation and adjustment potential of today's more advanced societies.

Is Africa facing an eco-Malthusian food crisis today?

While eco-Malthusian visions are not yet convincing for the world at large, they occasionally emerge as a popular way to understand the particular plight of Sub-Saharan Africa. In this region, the expansion of cropland area to boost food production, in order to keep pace with population growth, has led to serious environmental damage in the form of forest loss and habitat destruction. Damage to the cropland itself has also been severe, because population pressures on the land have led to reduced fallow times, less land recovery time between harvests, and hence a more rapid depletion of soil nutrients. This in turn has constrained food production. From 1990 to 2019, total food production per person in East Africa increased by only 1 percent. For Sub-Saharan Africa as a whole, UN estimates show that between 2001 and 2015, the share of Africa's population suffering from undernourishment fell from 26 percent to 18 percent, but this trend was subsequently reversed, and by 2019 the undernourished share increased again to 20 percent. Over that same time period, the population of Sub-Saharan Africa had grown from 683 million up to 1.11 billion, so the absolute number of those who were undernourished had increased by 44 million. Were it not for Africa's growing food imports, this number would have been much larger.

Africa's food problems are severe, yet they do not take the form of a classic Malthusian trap, in which population growth outstrips food production potential. This is because food production in Africa today is far below the known potential for the region. Most African farmers today use little or no fertilizer (only one-tenth as much per acre as farmers in Europe use), and only 5 percent of their cropland has been irrigated. Also, most of the cropped area in Africa is not yet sown with seeds improved through scientific plant breeding. As a consequence, average cereal crop yields per acre in Africa are only about one-fifth as high as in the developed world. Africa is failing to keep up with population growth not because it has exhausted its natural resource potential but instead because too little has been invested in developing that potential. Typically in Africa today, governments spend only about 5 percent of their budget on any kind of agricultural improvements, even though half of their citizens may depend on the farming sector for income and employment. If food production fails to keep up because nobody invests to make farms more productive, that qualifies as an acute public policy crisis, but it is not a classic Malthusian crisis.

Do Malthusians try to reduce population growth?

Thomas Malthus, in his day, never put much stock in efforts to control fertility. By the 20th century, however, public and private interventions to encourage "family planning" were commonplace in the industrial world, where births per woman were rapidly declining anyway. So it naturally became popular among modern-day Malthusians to advocate policy interventions to bring down fertility in developing countries as well. In 1974, at a UN World Population Conference in Bucharest, rich country governments told poor countries that they should slow population growth. The poor countries replied that what they really needed was more rapid economic growth.

International advocacy for aggressive family planning programs in the developing world fell out of favor later in the 1970s, after China's coercive one-child family policies led to female infants being killed by parents who wanted their one child to be a son, and when a state-sponsored sterilization policy in India led to explosive social tensions between Hindus and Muslims. In the decade between the 1974 World Population Conference in Bucharest and the 1984 International Conference on Population in Mexico City, favored approaches within the international assistance community shifted from rigid "supply-side" efforts to bring down fertility (e.g., giving men and women access to modern contraception) to a new "demand-side" approach that focused on reducing the desire for more births. This demand-side approach was advanced through an emphasis on increased child survival and a promotion of education and employment opportunities for girls and young women.

Aggressive supply-side efforts to limit fertility also came under attack from the Christian Right in America in the 1980s, as one part of a backlash against the 1973 *Roe v. Wade* Supreme Court decision that had decriminalized abortion. Abortion opponents at that time were losing the means to dictate policy inside the United States (*Roe v. Wade* would not be reversed until 2022) but they did manage, initially under the presidency of Ronald Reagan, to place tighter restrictions on programs supporting family planning abroad. Advocates who continue to favor family planning assistance today tend to emphasize human rights arguments—the rights of women to control their own fertility—rather than Malthusian arguments about scarce resources.

Do Malthusians argue that we should reduce food consumption?

Among those worried about food scarcity who no longer wish to promote fertility control, one alternative is a call for reduced food consumption per capita. This argument was first popularized in 1971, by a food activist named Frances Moore Lappé, who wrote a widely influential book (over 3 million copies sold) titled *Diet for a Small Planet*. The book argued that meat consumption in rich countries was using up scarce land resources to grow grain to feed chickens, pigs, and cattle, when grain should instead be used to prevent starvation in poor countries. Lappé argued against beef consumption in particular, observing that the protein beef cattle consumed in feed was 21 times greater than the amount that they finally made available in their meat for human consumption. On our "small planet" with limited resources, perhaps the only way to feed our growing numbers would be a move toward vegetarian diets.

Reducing meat consumption in rich countries today would certainly be good for both human health and the environment in those countries, and it would slow the accumulation of greenhouse gas (especially methane) in the atmosphere, but it would have only a limited impact on the food supplies available in poor countries. The International Food Policy Research Institute used a computer model of global agricultural markets to estimate the reduction in world hunger that might result from a 50 percent cut in per capita meat consumption from current levels in all high-income countries. Even under this extreme (and extremely unlikely) scenario, the reduction in child hunger in poor countries would only be one-half of 1 percent. The reason is that meat consumption in rich countries is mostly a result of agricultural resource use inside those same rich countries, not in places like Africa or South Asia where most hungry people reside. If rich countries ate less meat, citizen health would improve and greenhouse gas emissions would decline, but the major change in food markets would be an immediate reduction in total animal and crop production in those same rich countries, not an increase in food production or consumption in poor countries.

In much of Africa, meanwhile, becoming a vegetarian is not an option. On many dry lands in Africa, there is not enough rainfall to grow cereal crops, so the only source of food may be grass-fed animals, such as goats and cattle.

3

THE POLITICS OF INTERNATIONAL FOOD PRICES

What are "international" food prices?

International food prices are the prices of foods available for export into the world market. These prices will differ depending on the place of export. For example, in 2021 the price per ton (free on board, or FOB) of long grain rice was almost twice as high at export terminals in the United States as it was at export terminals in India. Also, the final price paid by the importer will be higher than this FOB price, because of the added costs of shipping and insurance.

Most important, the prices of foods in international markets at the border will usually differ from food prices in domestic markets "behind the border." Sometimes this is because governments add a tariff (a border tax) onto imported food. Sometimes this is because governments manipulate the value of their national currencies relative to the foreign currencies used when calculating international prices. In national politics, domestic food prices are usually more important than international prices, because these are the prices seen by domestic consumers, and because most food consumption around the world continues to depend on supplies produced by domestic farmers rather than supplies imported from abroad. Yet when a sudden or extreme increase in international food prices is encountered, this can trigger fears of a global food shortage—often dubbed a "global food crisis."

For example, high international food prices became an intense political issue in 2007–2008, when international market prices for rice, wheat, and corn all spiked sharply upward at the same time. By April 2008, the price of maize (corn) available for export had doubled compared to two years earlier; rice prices had tripled in just three months; and wheat reached its highest price in 28 years. Riots broke out in a number of developing countries that depended heavily on imported food, and it seemed that hunger was certain to increase as well. The *New York Times*, in a lead editorial, declared these surprising changes a "world food crisis." Robert Zoellick, president of the World Bank, warned that high food prices were particularly dangerous for the poor, who must spend half to three-quarters of their income on food. "There is no margin for survival," he said.

A global financial crisis in 2009 burst the inflationary bubble and caused these high international food prices to fall, but then in 2010 wheat prices increased sharply once more, following a heat wave and drought in Russia. Just as this second food price spike seemed to be passing by early 2012, a severe summer drought in the United States sent international corn prices spiking upward yet again.

This unusual series of international food price spikes between 2007 and 2012 momentarily transformed global expectations and debates around food. The price spikes were not just disruptive on their own terms; they called into question what had been a comforting assumption among most economists, that over the long term agricultural commodity prices would fall rather than rise, due to continued farm productivity gains.

What caused the 2007–2012 spikes in international food prices?

The cause of these disruptive international price spikes was widely misunderstood at the time. In retrospect, the most powerful explanation was not a sudden shortage of food overall, but instead just a shortage of food available for export, due to simultaneous changes in the trade policies of food-exporting countries. When food prices started to rise behind the border in domestic markets after 2006, numerous states began to restrict exports, hoping to keep their own domestic prices low. If enough big exporters do this at the same time, less food will be available for export so international prices will spike upward.

Export bans were the central problem, but critics feared that other factors had also played a role. Higher fuel costs (the price of petroleum was also spiking in 2008) were leading to an increase in biofuel production, such as ethanol from corn. This led to fears that fuel demands in rich countries were contributing to higher food prices and more hunger in poor countries.

Other critics faulted speculative behavior on the part of international investors, who were moving their money into commodity markets (pushing up not just food and fuel prices but metal prices as well) because of bursting investment bubbles in stock markets and real estate. In 2000, President Clinton had signed the Commodity Futures Modernization Act that reduced regulations governing the buying and selling of commodity futures by banks and securities firms. This opened the way for much more speculative buying and selling of food commodities. The volume of these trades did increase sharply after 2006, with impacts on the spot market price, but the futures contracts purchased by investors expire quickly, and only 2 percent of futures trades ever result in an actual delivery of goods, so speculative behavior in futures markets seems an unlikely foundation for longer-term international price trends.

One factor that cannot be blamed for this "global food crisis" was a slowdown in food production or in the growth of agricultural productivity. According to calculations from the US Department of Agriculture, the annual rate of growth of total factor productivity in agriculture, in both North America and Asia, was significantly higher in the 15 years up to 2007 than it had been in the two decades prior to that period. Nor were physical food shortages a cause of the 2008 price spike.

Rice prices tripled on the world market in 2008, but global rice production had actually grown more rapidly than consumption during the previous year, causing an increase in surplus stocks. Another explanation that could be dismissed was import demands by China. Rapid income growth was driving up China's demand for food, but China's own production was also increasing, and China was actually a net exporter of rice, wheat, and corn when international prices were spiking in 2007–2008.

The single biggest driver of international food price spikes in 2007–2008 and in 2010–2011 was government policy restraints on exports, and panic buying due to fears of such restraints. In 2007, economic growth in Asia had been high, fuel prices were up, and inflation fears were on the rise. At this point, a number of countries decided to place restrictions on agricultural exports, to protect their consumers at home from food price inflation. China imposed export taxes on grains and grain products. Argentina raised export taxes on wheat, corn, and soybeans. Russia raised export taxes on wheat. Malaysia and Indonesia imposed export taxes on palm oil. Egypt, Cambodia, Vietnam, and Indonesia eventually banned exports of rice. India, the world's third-largest rice exporter, banned exports of rice other than basmati.

When these export bans were instituted, international prices began spiking upward, which led importers to panic and to begin buying as much as they could before the price went even higher. This of course worsened the price spike. Media reports of shortages proliferated, and panic buying even spread to the United States, where frightened consumers descended on stores to buy rice. In April 2008, the Costco Wholesale Corporation and Walmart's Sam's Club had to limit sales of rice to four bags per customer per visit.

Memories of the 2008 export bans were still fresh in 2010, when a severe summer drought damaged grain production in Russia. Fearing a possible Russian export ban, importers accelerated their normal wheat purchases, which pushed the international price upward. This in turn pushed bread prices inside Russia to unacceptable levels, so in midsummer the government announced a temporary ban on all grain exports, a ban that kept international prices high for the next nine months.

The price spike of 2012 was less severe and was driven not by export bans but instead by an actual production shortfall, namely a severe drought that reduced total corn production in the United States by 13 percent. Higher corn prices became a serious short-term problem for livestock producers, and led to higher meat prices for consumers. Episodic production shortfalls of this kind had been seen before, and will probably be seen again. An earlier Midwest drought in 1988 had reduced US corn production by 31 percent.

How many people became hungry when international prices spiked in 2007–2008?

On this important issue experts disagree. While the crisis was under way, the World Bank produced a hasty estimate, based on a computer model, that said that the higher international food prices were pushing an added 100 million people around the world into poverty. The media carelessly reported this as an assertion that 100 million more people were going hungry. In the following year, the UN Food and Agriculture Organization (FAO) went even further, asserting that the number of under-nourished people worldwide had increased from 873 million in 2004–2006 up to 1.02 billion in 2009.

There were reasons from the start to be skeptical about the World Bank calculation. It was based on an artificial as-sumption that when international prices go up, national governments do not change their trade policies to offset the domestic impacts. In fact, trade policy changes such as export bans had produced the exaggerated international price spike in the first place. The FAO calculation was also suspect, because it was not made using a transparent method. Yet a consensus opinion in media and policy circles emerged that many more people had been made hungry, so the 1 billion number went essentially unchallenged.

Several years later, after the panic had passed, the FAO decided to reexamine its estimates, and in 2012 it published a remarkable revision. It adjusted its estimate for 2004–2006 upward, from 873 million to 898 million, and its estimate for 2007–2009 downward. It now asserted that the numbers of undernourished people in the world had actually *fallen* in 2007–2009, during the first peak of the crisis, down to 867 million, and had remained near that lower level in 2010–2012, despite continued high international prices and despite continued global population growth. These estimates implied that before, during, and after the peak of the crisis, the percentage of the world's population that was undernourished had actually fallen from 14 percent down to 13 percent, and finally down to just 12 percent in 2010–2012.

We can learn from these strangely revised FAO estimates that all such calculations are partly guesswork, and that using international food prices as a basis for estimating hunger is fundamentally unsound. This is because most of the world's poorest people, those most vulnerable to hunger, are not well connected to international food markets. In poor rural Africa, in contrast to more prosperous urban Africa, nearly all food remains local or homegrown, and it often consists of products seldom traded on the international market, such as goat meat, cassava, yams, and millet. Rural road systems in these countries are so poor and transport costs so high that international price transmission into the countryside is always weak. In South Asia, where the world's largest number of hungry people still live, national governments have long used trade restrictions to protect their domestic food markets from international price fluctuations. In 2011, for this reason, when the price of wheat was soaring on the world market, wheat flour prices in India, on the streets of New Delhi, were actually falling.

Spikes in international food prices do create serious economic hardship for urban consumers in countries that have allowed themselves to become significantly dependent on food imports, including many in the Caribbean, Central America, North Africa, and West Africa. These urban dwellers are generally better fed than the rural poor, but a sudden need to spend more for food will mean having less to spend on clothing, shelter, schooling, and other services. Food price increases that are temporary may not produce much in the way of actual undernutrition, but they will immediately generate social and political unrest. Even if they do not lead to hunger, they will be certain to lead to anger, and urban anger is typically more dangerous to governments than rural hunger. It will become a serious political problem even if most consumers are still getting the food they need.

Do international food price spikes cause violent conflict?

The international food price spikes of 2007–2008 and 2010–2011 were widely cited for triggering patterns of domestic social and political unrest. The 2007–2008 price event coincided with street protests or riots in Burkina Faso, Cameroon, Senegal, Mauritania, Côte d'Ivoire, Egypt, Morocco, Haiti, Mexico, Bolivia, Yemen, Uzbekistan, Bangladesh, Pakistan, Sri Lanka, and South Africa. In Haiti, food riots caused the death of five people and led to dismissal of the prime minister. Five protesters were also killed in Somalia. In Cameroon, at least 24 people were killed in the worst unrest in 15 years. In Pakistan, the army was deployed to stop the theft of food from fields and warehouses. When international wheat prices then respiked in the winter of 2010–2011, street demonstrations began in North Africa, where wheat flour, used for bread, is a basic staple. During the course of this "Arab Spring," governments were toppled in Tunisia, Libya, and Egypt.

Some analysts concluded, from these events, that international food price spikes had become a dominant new cause of social unrest and violent conflict around the world. When the third price spike began in 2012, driven this time by a US drought, one respected academic warned, in a news interview, "We are on the verge of another crisis, the third in five years, and likely to be the worst yet, capable of causing new food riots and turmoil on a par with the Arab Spring." Fortunately, this didn't happen.

In retrospect, the Arab Spring was a political upheaval that emerged from far more than just food prices. In Tunisia, where the protests began in December 2010, the people who took to the streets were not demanding cheaper bread. Instead they were calling for dignity, the removal of a corrupt government, and more jobs. The crisis began when a young man took his own life not to protest high food prices but instead to protest an insult from an arrogant government official. When the protests in Tunisia brought the government down, equally restless urban dwellers seeking political change in Libya and Egypt saw their opportunity and took to the streets for the same purpose. These urban dwellers in North Africa were not "hungry." In Cairo, the price of bread had been held low by government subsidies for so long that average daily calorie intake was at European levels, and diseases linked to obesity were a growing problem.

Have higher food prices triggered "land grabs" in Africa?

As would be expected, the higher international food prices seen after 2007 triggered larger investments in agricultural production worldwide, including the purchase or rental of underutilized farmland. Many investors—including private firms and sovereign wealth funds from China, India, South Korea, and oil-rich states in the Persian Gulf—saw land in Africa as potentially useful for the production of both food and biofuels. Because most agricultural land in Africa was legally under the control of governments rather than individual farmers (only about 10 percent of land in Africa was formally tenured), foreign investors began approaching African governments, including less scrupulous local officials, with offers to lease substantial areas of farming land. Between October 2008 and August 2009 alone, over 115 million acres of farmland acquisitions were announced.

The obvious risk with such land deals is that the local farming or herding populations currently on the land will be uncompensated for any resulting disruption or destruction of their livelihood. If their land is taken over by investors for mechanized crop farming, or for plantation-style biofuels production, they will run the risk of being displaced. Social justice non-governmental organizations (NGOs) were quick to brand this new wave of investments a "land grab," and to demand stronger protection for local communities.

The land grab terminology was apt, but in most cases it was not foreigners grabbing land directly from African farmers; instead it was African governments and government officials grabbing the land from their own citizens, then making a profit by selling or leasing it to foreigners. Africans saw what was going on and some protested. In Madagascar in 2009, violent street demonstrations broke out over a government plan to lease 3.2 million acres of land to a South Korean corporation, Daewoo, to produce corn and palm oil. The government was replaced, and the plan was dropped.

When the FAO studied these issues in 2012, it observed that despite many wild claims about land grabs in Africa, there was very little reliable data. Second, it saw that in many cases domestic investors had acquired more land than foreigners. Third, the implications for local farmers were seen to depend largely on the crop production systems selected by the investor. If an investor brings in new technology and infrastructure and makes contracted purchases from local farmers, there may be benefits for the rural poor.

Why did international food prices spike again in 2021–2022?

International food prices fell back down after 2012, as panic over opportunities to import subsided and when most countries lifted their bans on exports. By 2015, prices had returned to the level of the 1980s, where they remained until 2020, when they spiked up again. By August 2021 they had climbed in real terms (discounted for inflation) back to the high level of 2011. This increase was indirectly triggered by the onset of the global COVID-19 pandemic.

Economic lockdowns imposed in response to COVID-19 immediately disrupted both the production and transport of food, driving up domestic prices and leading to panic buying. The higher domestic prices then triggered a resumption of national export bans, stabilizing some domestic markets but driving international prices higher still. As of mid-June 2020, 23 different countries had implemented a total of 104 prohibitions on agrifood exports, sometimes to include export bans on fertilizers as well. This brought back a level of export restrictions on food not seen since 2012.

This response to COVID-19 was doing damage even before Russia's shocking invasion of Ukraine in February 2022, an event that triggered additional export bans and drove up international wheat prices by an additional 34 percent. Russia, the world's number two exporter of wheat with a 17.5 percent market share, announced a ban on its own exports of wheat and other grains in March, a move followed by Ukraine itself, plus Egypt, India, Kazakhstan, Kosovo, and Serbia. By June, 22 countries around the world were restricting wheat exports, covering more than one-fifth of global trade. Ukraine's ports on the Black Sea were also blockaded early in the war, sharply cutting that nation's exports of corn, barley, and sunflower seeds.

In this new context, Secretary-General of the UN António Guterres warned in June 2022 that the world was now facing "an unprecedented global hunger crisis." He said the number of severely food insecure people around the world had doubled to 276 million, and warned that "this year's food access issues could become next year's global food shortage. No country will be immune to the social and economic repercussions of such a catastrophe." As was seen after the 2008 food crisis, however, even when export bans create a significant shortage of some foods available to buy on the world market, this does not always shrink domestic supplies, and it is certainly not the same thing as a global food shortage.

After Ukraine and Russia reached an agreement (brokered by Turkey) in July 2022 to allow a resumption of agricultural product exports from some Black Sea ports, a bit of optimism returned. By that time, international wheat and corn prices had already fallen back to their pre-invasion level, yet they were still 50 percent higher than they had been 30 months earlier, and there was no guarantee against a resumed blockage as long as the war continued.

In some cases, this renewal of high international food prices after 2019 did bring real hunger, but usually owing to other misfortunes. Lebanon was hard-hit, because wheat accounted for 38 percent of that nation's total calorie consumption, and 80 percent of Lebanon's wheat had traditionally been imported, nearly all coming from Russia and Ukraine. Yet the new import price shock for wheat was made far worse by a financial collapse in Lebanon's banking sector in 2019, one that cut the nation's currency value by nearly 95 percent, driving consumer price inflation above 200 percent. This wider economic crisis, when compounded by the economic impacts of COVID-19, pushed three-quarters of Lebanon's population into poverty by the end of 2021, even before Russia invaded Ukraine. In 2022, the UN World Food Programme estimated that half of Lebanon's population was experiencing hunger.

What can we learn from longer trends in international food prices?

We have mostly learned that fluctuations in international food prices are not only hard to predict but also are widely misinterpreted by both the media and policymakers while they are under way. The distinction between international prices and domestic prices is frequently overlooked, along with the tendency for prices to be influenced by macroeconomic factors from beyond the food and farming sector.

Over most of the 20th century, international food commodity prices were in a fortunate decline, despite extremely rapid global population growth, thanks mostly to continuous gains in agricultural productivity. This longer-term decline was interrupted, however, during both world wars in the first half of that century and then by a remarkable interlude of global inflation in the 1970s. The international price of both wheat and corn suddenly doubled between 1971 and 1974, and when the price of soybeans rose so high that even the United States briefly imposed an export ban in 1973, *Time* magazine branded it a "world food crisis." *Time* claimed that hunger and famine were now ravaging "hundreds of millions of the poorest citizens in at least 40 nations."

This 1970s food price crisis had a number of characteristics similar to the subsequent 2008 price spike. Just as in 2008, the price of all commodities, not just food, was spiking upward, indicating a macroeconomic cause originating from beyond the food and farming sector. Once again, physical shortages around the world weren't driving prices; the world wasn't running out of all commodities at the same time.

The macroeconomic malfunction in the 1970s was inflationary growth, linked primarily to lax monetary policies by the Federal Reserve Board in the United States. There was a parallel here to the 2008 price spike, which also followed moves by the Fed to cut interest rates to record-low levels. And just as in 2008, the 1970s price spike was made worse by export restrictions. In addition to a temporary US embargo on soybean sales in 1973, Argentina, Brazil, Thailand, Myanmar (then Burma), and the EU (then the Common Market) restricted food exports, stabilizing prices at home but destabilizing international market prices. And just as in 2008, food riots broke out in urban neighborhoods in poor countries when prices spiked in the 1970s.

The price spikes of the 1970s were brought to an end by a decisive tightening of US monetary policy, which slowed economic growth worldwide and threw the US economy into a recession after 1981. When international food prices finally dropped after 1981, many interpreted this as the end of the "food crisis," but in fact a more genuine hunger crisis—one driven by lowered incomes in Africa and Latin America—was just beginning. Africa and Latin America are commodity-exporting regions, so they actually suffer when the price of oil, copper, and other exported commodities drops. More people actually became hungry in these regions *after* the international price of food fell, during the economic recession and the debt crisis years that followed.

High international commodity prices usually impose a relatively small sacrifice on food consumers in rich countries, because diets in these countries consist heavily of packaged and processed food products and restaurant meals, in which the final cost to consumers comes from many things other than farm commodities. In the United States, farm commodities now make up only 8 percent of final food costs to consumers. The cost of the corn in a box of cornflakes contributes less than 2 percent to the final cost to consumers. When consumers in rich countries do adjust to high international commodity prices, it is often through a temporary reduction in meat consumption, or a substitution of hamburger for steak, which is again not a huge sacrifice. When grain prices increase, the first adjustment rich countries make is to feed less corn and soybeans to farm animals such as chickens, pigs, and cattle. In 1974, when corn prices more than doubled, the United States reduced the feeding of grain to livestock by 25 percent, which freed up more grain for direct consumption as food. Herd sizes were cut, eventually leading to higher meat prices and a temporary reduction in meat consumption in wealthy societies.

Because international price fluctuations can be expected to continue, uncertain and even misguided conclusions about their link to human hunger will probably also continue to be drawn by the media and in the political arena. A better understanding of the more fundamental causes of human hunger around the world will be the focus of the next chapter.

4

THE POLITICS OF CHRONIC HUNGER AND FAMINE

How do we measure hunger?

In our personal lives, hunger is a sensation we feel regularly just before mealtime. In the world of politics and public policy, "hunger" is often used as a shorthand substitute for chronic undernutrition, a long-term condition that includes either a protein-energy deficit in the diet, a micronutrient deficit, or both. A protein-energy deficit occurs when the intake of calories falls consistently below the total energy the human body burns. A micronutrient deficit occurs when the body does not get enough critical vitamins or minerals, such as iron, zinc, iodine, or vitamin A.

The visible indications of a protein-energy deficit include stunting (a short height relative to age), wasting (a low weight relative to height), and underweight (a low weight relative to age). All these conditions can have serious medical consequences, particularly if they begin in the early months of life before age two. Inadequate early nutrition can lead to reduced cognition plus increased susceptibility to infectious disease, and it is a major cause of infant mortality. In the poorly fed regions of Africa, children under five die seven times as often as in the United States. Globally, these problems of chronic malnutrition are fortunately in retreat. In 2020, roughly

20 percent of children under five were affected by stunting, down from more than 30 percent in 2000.

When measuring children for height and weight, one complicating factor is that human stature and body size are influenced by genetics as well as nutrition, so small stature does not always reflect ill health; some children can be "small but healthy." Nonetheless, adverse long-term health effects have been confirmed statistically for populations in which large numbers of individuals are of below-average stature. Diets that provide abundant early access to protein, calcium, and vitamins A and D are known to improve health as well as stature. As diets have improved around the world, in fact, people have grown not just more healthy but taller as well. In the United States today, compared to a century ago, the average adult male is three inches taller and also enjoys a significantly longer life expectancy.

How many people around the world remain chronically undernourished?

Since 1974, the UN Food and Agriculture Organization (FAO) has been tasked with estimating the total number of chronically undernourished people worldwide. These estimates have been based on incomplete data, crude assumptions, and a methodology that sometimes changes, so they are often criticized for their variability and imprecision. The FAO traditionally generated its estimates country by country, based on rough calculations such as the total availability of food in each country, the demographic structure of the population, the distribution of food access within the population (calculated when possible from nationally representative household surveys), and an assumed level of daily dietary energy required to provide adequate nutrition. Using such methods, the UN estimated that at least 702 million and as many as 828 million people "faced hunger" in 2021. This condition affected roughly 30 percent of the population in East and Middle

Africa, 19 percent in West Africa, and 16 percent in South Asia and also in the Caribbean.

Globally, considerable progress has been made. The prevalence of undernourishment (PoU) has fallen from 36 percent in 1970, down to 16 percent in 1990, then down to 8 percent by 2013. That level remained virtually unchanged up through 2019, but then climbed to around 9.9 percent in 2020 and 9.8 percent in 2021. Much of this increase after 2019 reflected impacts from the global COVID-19 pandemic.

These crude estimates of global hunger tend to underestimate micronutrient deficiencies, which are called "hidden hunger" because they are so often unseen. For example, a lack of iron in the diet leads to anemia, which tends to escape direct observation but can reduce cognitive and physical capacities and is associated with reduced economic productivity and increased mortality. Among women of reproductive age, anemia can lead to stillbirth, low birth weight, and infant mortality. The World Health Organization (WHO) estimates that in 82 low- and middle-income (LMICs) countries, overall anemia prevalence among women of reproductive age stood at 31.6 percent in 2018, which was down from 35.6 percent in 2000 but still much too high. In India, and in some West African countries, anemia prevalence was closer to 50 percent.

In some countries, severe undernutrition can persist in the countryside while chronic disease problems linked to excessive food consumption are worsening in urban areas, creating a so-called double burden of malnutrition. When micronutrient deficits are also present it can even be described as a "triple burden." Different forms of malnutrition can be found within a single community, or even within a single household (e.g., if male children are given more to eat than female children).

How is food insecurity different from chronic undernutrition?

Beyond traditional measures of chronic undernourishment, the UN now also measures something it calls food insecurity.

People are described as food insecure if they "lack regular access to enough safe and nutritious food for normal growth and development and an active and healthy life." Food insecurity is measured through individual surveys, by asking people, for example, if at any time over the previous 12 months they ever worried about not having enough food to eat, or ate only a few kinds of foods, or had to skip a meal, or went without eating for a whole day. Depending on the number of "yes" answers, individuals can be described as having mild, moderate, or severe food insecurity.

Measurements of food insecurity such as these are derived through more transparent methods, and they can be applied at an individual or local level, not just nationally, but they rely on human memory and they mix psychological with behavioral variables. By asking if something happened or was experienced *at any time over a previous year*, these surveys also tend to generate a higher estimate of "hungry" (severely food insecure) people. The UN estimated that 924 million people, or 11.7 percent of the global population, experienced severe food insecurity in 2021.

What causes chronic undernutrition?

Chronic undernutrition, the UN's traditional measure of hunger, primarily reflects a persistence of deep poverty, and it usually goes away when poverty goes away. Fortunately, the prevalence of poverty around the world has been in a long-term decline. In the second half of the 20th century, as Steven Pinker has shown, the share of the world's citizens living in extreme poverty (considered now to be those living on less than $1.90 per person a day) fell sharply from 60 percent down to 10 percent. By 2015, this share had fallen to just 8 percent. This decline was temporarily reversed by the economic shutdowns and job losses during the COVID-19 pandemic beginning in 2020, which temporarily pushed an estimated 75 to 95 million people back into poverty.

Not all of those living in poverty are hungry, but the vast majority of those around the world with chronic hunger are poor. The World Bank has calculated that 78 percent of the world's poorest people live in rural areas and rely largely on farming, livestock, aquaculture, and other agricultural work to make a living and put food on their plates. When these poor farmers and farm laborers can't afford to buy the food they need or can't afford to buy the materials needed to produce their own food, they will experience chronic undernutrition. In the countryside this is commonly a seasonal condition that sets in if the food supplies previously harvested begin to run out before a next crop is ready to harvest, initiating a period known as the "hunger season."

Other risk factors for chronic undernutrition include having fewer years of schooling and suffering from low social status and political marginalization. Other things being equal, ethnic minorities are more likely to be hungry. For example, in Sri Lanka, Indian Tamils are at a disadvantage. In Central America, stunting is twice as widespread among indigenous children compared to non-indigenous children, and in South Asia, hill tribes and "scheduled castes" suffer greater nutrition deficits than others. In Africa, female-headed households are more at risk. The least well-fed individuals in many societies are orphans and street children.

Poverty may seem highly visible to outsiders visiting cities in low-income countries, but it is poverty in the countryside that usually generates the larger share of chronic undernutrition. There are roughly twice as many poor and hungry people in the African countryside compared to urban areas, and in South Asia the ratio is three to one. This greater prevalence of hunger in rural areas reflects a cruel paradox: rural dwellers typically work in farming for a living, yet they often fail to get enough food for their own needs. This is because in South Asia and Africa many rural dwellers are either landless agricultural laborers, working only seasonally and for low pay, or they are impoverished smallholder farmers who have access to land but lack the tools needed (irrigation, improved seeds, fertilizers) to make their farm labor productive. They are hard-working, frugal, and they waste nothing, but the food and money often run out before the next harvest. They are living in what development economists call a "poverty trap."

Does chronic hunger trigger political unrest?

Food price spikes can cause social protests and even riots, but chronic hunger by itself is seldom a trigger for political un-rest. It should be, but it is not. Persistently poor and hungry communities seldom have the means to make trouble or threaten governments. A preponderance of the hungry are usually young children or illiterate women located in remote rural settings, lacking in political knowledge or the means to organize. Often they will be from disadvantaged castes or from marginalized racial and ethnic groups. They may also be living under a nondemocratic political regime led by a single ruling party, a single dynastic family, the military, or a theocracy of religious clerics who do not wish to share their power. In sys-tems such as these, governments that ignore poor and hungry people in the countryside often get away with it.

As mentioned in Chapter 3, physical hunger and undernutrition were not the cause of the "Arab Spring" street demonstrations that toppled governments in Tunisia, Libya, and Egypt in 2011. In urban Tunisia, where the demonstrations began (over issues of government corruption, unemployment, and personal dignity), chronic undernutrition was hard to find. In all of Tunisia, only 2.9 percent of children under five were underweight, less than one-fifth of the global average of 16.2 percent. In fact, none of the food protests of 2008 and none of the Arab Spring protests of 2011 broke out in a country that had fallen into an "extremely alarming" global hunger index category as measured by the International Food Policy Research Institute. If physical hunger were a leading source of political instability, it would be rural rather than urban populations leading the demonstrations, and governments (to ensure their survival) would be investing far more in rural agricultural development.

Is chronic undernutrition a problem in the United States?

In the United States, the number one dietary health problem today is chronic disease linked to obesity, not undernutrition. In 2019, 42 percent of American adults were clinically obese. This represents a dramatic change from the middle years of the 20th century, when only 10 percent of Americans were obese, and when deep poverty in regions like Appalachia or the Mississippi Delta generated widespread undernutrition. The United States today still has too many communities living in poverty, but today's poor are far less likely to suffer from a protein-energy deficit.

One full century ago, when average consumer income in the United States was only one-fourth as high as today, and when the price of most basic food commodities was twice as high in real terms, getting enough to eat was a serious problem for large parts of the population. At the beginning of the 20th century, the average American spent 41 percent of disposable personal income on food (four times the level of today), and low-income Americans often could not afford a healthy diet. During the hard times of the Great Depression in the 1930s, several thousand Americans died each year from diseases such as pellagra (niacin deficiency), beriberi (thiamin deficiency), rickets (vitamin D deficiency), and scurvy (vitamin C deficiency). In 1938, over 20 percent of preschool children in America had rickets, with hundreds dying from this disabling ailment.

During the second half of the 20th century, dietary deficits such as these were steadily overcome thanks to a decline in absolute poverty, a continued decline in food commodity prices, and an expanding set of government-funded anti-hunger interventions. Congress passed the National School Lunch Act in 1946, partly in reaction to the poor nutritional status that had been discovered among young men drafted into military service early in World War II. Then in the 1970s, following media reports of scandalous poverty and hunger in rural Appalachia, a federal food stamp program, which provided food purchase credits to low-income families, was dramatically expanded, and a Special Supplemental Nutrition Program for Women, Infants, and Children (the WIC program) was created to improve the health of low-income pregnant women, new mothers, infants, and young children at nutritional risk. Food stamp spending quadrupled between 1970 and 1973 alone, and participation in the program increased from 4 million in 1970, up to 15 million by 1974, and 22.4 million by 1981. The program then continued to expand, and by 2021 it was serving 41 million Americans.

These federal food assistance programs have produced gratifying results. Since the 1990s, the US Department of Agriculture has conducted annual surveys to measure different degrees of "food insecurity" at the household level, ranging from zero insecurity all the way up to a condition of insecurity with actual "hunger." By the time these surveys began in 1995, they showed that only 4.1 percent of American households were food insecure "with hunger" (a category later relabeled "very low food security").

This strong gain against hunger has been sustained, although at an expanding cost to taxpayers in recent years. In 2007 the SNAP (food stamp) program delivered $30 billion worth of food purchase credits, then this cost increased to $78 billion in 2011, and to $135 billion in 2021 (partly due to increased benefits during the COVID pandemic, explained below). Families qualify for SNAP benefits depending primarily on their gross income level. In 2023 the monthly gross income level limit for a family of four in Georgia was $3,007.

Several program changes and expansions have been driving up SNAP budget costs. In 1996 the law was changed to allow individual states to ease the eligibility requirements and to make more aggressive efforts to enroll eligible residents, giving them a way to channel more federal money to their communities. A switch was also made late in the 1990s allowing benefits to be delivered through an EBT card that could be swiped discreetly at checkout, rather than through the redemption of paper coupons. This avoided public shaming and reduced the stigma associated with being a food stamp recipient. One result was a significant increase in participation rates. In 2001, only about half of those eligible participated, but by 2011, three-quarters of those eligible were receiving benefits.

The 2020 COVID-19 pandemic led to an even more dramatic increase in the use of SNAP. Many more Americans became eligible for benefits because they had lost work, and by 2022, 41 million Americans were participating. Monthly benefits were increased in response to the pandemic emergency, work requirements were lessened, and in 2021 the Department of Agriculture updated the Thrifty Food Plan it uses to calculate benefits, bringing an additional 18 percent increase in outlays. These measures were costly, but alongside private food charity efforts they helped minimize the experience of actual hunger during the pandemic. USDA surveys revealed that only 3.9 percent of households experienced "very low food security" at any given time in 2020, which was actually below the 4.1 percent that had reported this condition in the previous year before the pandemic. The next year's survey showed that the prevalence of very low food security during the 30-day period before December 2021 was only 2.2 percent.

For many SNAP recipients, a significant share of the food purchases made using program benefits would likely be made even without those benefits. Using SNAP benefits in place of personal income to buy food makes it possible for low-income households to allocate more cash to other things such as housing, clothing, health, and education. In this way, the SNAP program functions not just as food assistance but as an important income support and insurance program for the poor. When President Clinton signed legislation in 1996 to "end welfare as we know it," advocates for the poor realized they could replace some of the discontinued welfare payments by expanding the SNAP program, which is what they did. This evolution of the program beyond straight food assistance drew criticism from public welfare critics, but the critics find SNAP harder to criticize than straight welfare, because shrinking SNAP is seen as risking more hunger, which to most politicians is worse than just risking more poverty.

Advocacy groups continue to argue that hunger in America is a significant emergency. They do this by citing USDA's official survey data on "food insecurity," even though only "very low food security" is what USDA might consider hunger. The advocates know that most media reports will fail to make this distinction and use the terms interchangeably. The resulting exaggeration of America's hunger problems has made it more difficult for dietary health advocates to bring attention to the nation's larger problem of chronic disease caused by excess food consumption and obesity.

In 2022, for example, traditional anti-hunger advocates championed a White House Conference on Hunger, Nutrition, and Health. Advocates for dietary health had to fight hard to move the conversation beyond proposals to help more people purchase still more food—which would include foods with too much sugar, salt, and fat, since SNAP does not restrict such foods. The one-day conference did list reducing diet-related disease as one of its goals, but most of the specific proposals that emerged were projects to boost food purchasing power, such as raising the minimum wage to $15 per hour and expanding the Child Tax Credit.

Do developing countries have policy remedies for chronic undernutrition?

Many middle-income developing countries have also operated "safety net" programs for the poor designed to protect against undernutrition. One of the more successful was Brazil, where

President Lula da Silva launched a Zero Hunger (Fome Zero) program in January 2003. By 2006, according to the FAO, this program had reduced that nation's undernourished population from 17 million to 11.9 million. Achieving this success required multiple separate policy interventions, and a continuing outlay of significant budget resources.

Brazil's strategy initially included a $400 million conditional cash transfer program, called Food Cards, to supplement the income of poor families when buying more food (the cash transfers were conditioned on school attendance and health checkups); a $130 million program to purchase food from family farmers (PAA); a $65 million health and nutrition program for the elderly, children, and nursing mothers to address illnesses caused by vitamin and micronutrient deficiencies; an expanded school feeding program; a program to monitor food intake; a food and nutrition education program; and a food supply and distribution program targeting low-income populations in larger cities. In 2009, so-called Family Grants benefiting 12.4 million families replaced the original Food Cards, at a greatly expanded annual cost to the state of $6.5 billion. These Family Grants in 2009 represented 2 percent of Brazil's federal budget, but this was only 0.4 percent of GDP. Less prosperous countries are not able to afford such programs, and countries with less administrative capacity are not able to implement them properly.

Brazil's programs paid off in terms of improved health and nutrition outcomes. In the city of Guaribas, the Food Card program helped to end infant deaths attributable to malnutrition and to expand vaccine coverage from 9 to 96 percent and prenatal care from 10 to 80 percent. The Fome Zero program's biggest challenge was striking a balance between doing enough to reach all of the poor, versus doing so much as to discourage private investments in the delivery of market-based nutrition and health services. Local Management Committees helped ensure appropriate targeting of public assistance by scrutinizing local Cadastro Unico (Unified Registers) of those in extreme poverty.

Governments elsewhere in the developing world have implemented food subsidy programs that are less well administered or less well targeted. One approach has been to set up parallel food supply systems for the poor in which citizens holding ration cards can go to "fair price shops" to purchase cheap bread or flour. India has operated such a system for decades, but management is poor and waste and corruption have been rampant. Another approach is to flood urban markets with government-purchased grain, a method often used to excess in Egypt. This approach is costly to the government, it makes food artificially cheap for all urban dwellers, not just the poor, and it often fails to reach rural areas where needs are greatest. Food safety net programs are nominally intended to improve nutrition, but their deeper motivation is also to deliver benefits to politically powerful urban groups supporting the government, such as civil servants, policemen, and labor unions.

Micronutrient deficits can also be addressed by policy interventions, often through the "fortification" of wheat flour with iron, folic acid, or vitamin B, usually at centralized industrial milling facilities. This is a relatively inexpensive process (it adds only a tiny fraction of a penny to the cost of a loaf of bread) and it is effective for those who get the fortified flour, but once again it can exclude the rural economy, where milling is small-scale and localized. An alternative fortification approach is biofortification, achieved by selectively breeding crop seeds with a higher zinc, iron, or beta carotene content. Scientists working for international research centers have successfully developed varieties of maize and sweet potato for Africa that have orange rather than white flesh, to deliver more vitamin A to protect against blindness.

Supporting broadly based income growth has always been the best long-run approach for reducing chronic undernutrition in developing countries. In the poorest agricultural societies, in Asia and Africa, this requires in the first instance an increase in the productivity of small farmers.

More than 2 billion people live and work on about 550 million small farms in these regions, and 40 percent of them live on incomes of less than US $2 per day. So long as agricultural labor earns only this much, the vast majority of rural citizens who work as farmers will remain poor and hence vulnerable to chronic undernutrition. Rural poverty and hunger worsened in Sub-Saharan Africa in the 1980s and 1990s largely because the average annual value added from farm labor was low and actually falling (from $418 in 1980, to just $379 by 1997). Meanwhile in East Asia, hunger was declining because average value added per farm worker was increasing sharply, up by 50 percent in Thailand and up by 100 percent in China. Increasing the productivity of farm labor typically requires the introduction of new technologies such as improved seeds, fertilizers, and machinery. It also requires government investment in basic rural public goods such as roads and electricity. Because governments in Africa have made few such investments, farm productivity remains low and large numbers remain poor and hungry.

What is the difference between undernutrition and famine?

A famine takes place when large numbers of people die quickly in a specific location because they have not had enough food to eat. Some die from actual starvation—acute wasting—while others die from diseases that attack people who are in a weakened state.

The UN officially declares a famine based on three criteria: at least 20 percent of households in an area must face extreme food shortages and a limited ability to cope; the acute malnutrition rate must exceed 30 percent; and the death rate must exceed two persons per day per 10,000 people in the population. While low food intake still afflicts hundreds of millions of poor people in the developing world, actual famines have fortunately become rare. Small famines still take place, and larger future famines are always possible, but in the second decade of the 21st century, famine deaths relative to our much larger total number of people on earth fell close to zero.

When have famines taken place?

Famine is as old as recorded history. In the book of Revelation, famine is represented as one of the four horsemen of the Apocalypse. Europe suffered a great famine in 1315–1317 that killed millions. In France during the Hundred Years' War (1337–1453), a combination of warfare, crop failures, and epidemics reduced the population by two-thirds. In Ireland in 1845–1849, famine triggered by a recurring potato blight killed 1 million people outright and drove another million from the country as refugees. In India, there were 14 famines between the 11th and 17th centuries, and India's great famine of 1876–1878 killed 6 to 10 million people.

By the 20th century, famine had largely disappeared from western Europe, but it continued to appear in Asia, Africa, and also in eastern Europe. In the Soviet Union under Lenin and Stalin, the Ukraine experienced one famine in 1921–1922, and a second, more severe, in 1932–1933. During World War II, the city of Leningrad suffered a famine that killed roughly 1 million people. In Asia, a famine visited Bengal in 1943, killing 1.5 million to 3 million people. Starvation devastated China in 1958–1961, during Mao Zedong's disastrous Great Leap Forward, killing as many as 30 million people, the single largest famine of all time. A famine began in North Korea in 1996, and continued for a time to a lesser extent, with a death toll impossible for outsiders to estimate given the closed nature of that state. In Africa, famine struck in the Sahel and in Ethiopia in the early 1970s and then again in Ethiopia and Sudan in the 1980s. More recently, famines were formally declared in southern Somalia in 2011 and South Sudan in 2017. In 2021, famines probably took place amid civil war in both Yemen and Ethiopia, but UN officials did not have sufficient access to the suffering regions to make a formal famine declaration.

What causes famines?

Famines have diverse causes. In some instances, a natural event may be the trigger, such as the drought in the African Sahel in the early 1970s that devastated both grain production and the forage needed for animals. In other cases (Ireland in 1845), a crop disease—in this case, a potato blight—can wipe out staple food production. In still other cases, such as Bangladesh in 1974, it can be rain-induced flooding, which disrupts agricultural production and drives food prices in the market beyond the reach of the poor. In Ethiopia, Sudan, and Mozambique in the 1980s, adverse impacts from drought were compounded by violent internal conflicts. In the Russian city of Leningrad in 1941, famine broke out when a surrounding German army intentionally blocked access to relief.

Ideology also can cause famine. In Ukraine in 1932–1933, Stalin took land and food away from private farmers because he viewed them as "capitalist" enemies of the working class. There was no drought, no blight, no flood, and no war—just a coercive government takeover intended to "socialize" the farming sector. Peasants who resisted were imprisoned or shot. Production fell, but forcible state procurements of grain continued, and at least 6 million people starved in one of the richest grain-growing regions of the world. More than ideological blindness may have been at work; historian Robert Conquest, author of *Harvest of Sorrow*, depicted these events as a "terror famine," an intentional campaign to starve Ukrainians suspected of political disloyalty to Moscow.

The famine in China in 1959–1961 was also driven by ideology—in this case, a 1958 decision by Mao Zedong to organize food production (and everything else) according to a system of people's communes. Ownership of farmland and control over grain harvests were both taken away, which eliminated any incentive for farmers to be productive. Peasant farmers also had their labor burdened by a new requirement that they begin producing steel out of scrap metal in "backyard furnaces." When grain production collapsed in 1959, requirements by local Communist Party cadres to deliver grain to the state to feed the urban workforce were nonetheless increased. This left the peasants with nothing for themselves, and 15 to 30 million starved. Mao was finally forced to abandon most of the policies that were causing the famine in 1962, and once he did the famine ended.

Despite this wide variety of famine causes, some scholars have tried to offer more generalized explanations. The most prominent modern famine scholar is Amartya Sen, a Bengali economist and philosopher who won a Nobel Prize in 1998 for his contribution to welfare economics. Sen, who witnessed the famine in Bengal in 1943 as a young boy, wrote an important book in 1981 (*Poverty and Famines: An Essay on Entitlement and Deprivation*) challenging the conventional belief that famines are caused by "food availability declines." Sen had found that during the 1943 Bengal famine, locally available food supplies did not decline; the deprivation resulted instead from a surge in wartime spending by Great Britain, the colonial power in control of Bengal, threatened by the army of Japan at the time. British spending increased urban food purchases, which sucked rice out of the countryside, leaving rural dwellers with no affordable food. As many as 3 million died, even though the total quantity of food available had never declined.

Sen explains a 1974 Bangladesh famine in much the same way. Floods disrupted agricultural employment, which in turn cut the income of landless farmworkers. The floods also created an *expectation* of rice shortages, which caused hoarding and panic buying, finally driving prices out of reach of the poor. Vulnerable groups that depended on a particular relationship between the market value of their own labor and the market price of rice found that their *exchange entitlement* (Sen's terminology) to food had been taken away. Those with a more direct entitlement to food—for example, those owning the land that produced the food—did not starve.

Sen's warnings of famine dangers linked to unregulated markets remain popular, yet his own later work shifted its emphasis to a concern regarding undemocratic political systems. Sen observed that famines do not tend to occur in democratic political systems, where leaders know they will be punished in the next election if they allow their own people to starve. Democratic India avoided famine in 1965 and 1966, despite two consecutive years of failing monsoon rains, because the leadership turned to the outside world for millions of tons of emergency food aid and then expanded its public food distribution system. Nondemocratic China provided no such response when the Great Leap failed, and it even covered up its famine from the outside world. It is the states lacking both free elections and free markets—such as China under Mao, or subsequently North Korea—that will be the most famine-prone.

How do famines end?

Famines can end for nearly as many different reasons as they begin. In the case of Ireland, famine deaths eventually declined in part because so many fled the country (including a large emigration to the United States) and also because so many potential victims had already died. In addition, Britain finally responded by sending food and funds to help Ireland, so by 1849–1850, public workhouses were able to care for those left destitute by the continuing crop failures.

In the case of Ukraine in 1933, roughly 25 percent of the population eventually perished, including nearly all of the propertied farmers who had resisted the move toward socialized agriculture. Once private agriculture had been destroyed and Stalin's political objectives achieved, he reduced mandatory state procurements from the region and allowed food distribution to resume, so the famine subsided. In the case of the Bengal famine of 1943, the crisis ended when the government in London finally accepted the need to import 1 million tons of grain to Bengal, to discourage hoarding and bring food prices back down to a level the poor could afford. In the case of Mao's famine in China, the abandonment of the Great Leap policies, a decision to permit grain imports, and a reduction in mandatory state procurements were all key to ending the starvation. In the case of the African Sahel, surviving pastoralist populations first relocated southward to less drought-prone regions, and then, fortunately, the cyclical rains improved. In the case of Ethiopia, Sudan, and Mozambique in the 1980s, famines that were largely triggered by drought and civil conflict ended when the rains returned or the civil conflicts diminished.

What has been the most successful international response to famine?

The best international response to famine is to bring in food and medical aid from the outside—but not too soon and not for too long. If international food aid is distributed too soon, at feeding stations in rural market towns after a drought, some people who are not yet starving will be tempted to leave their farms and relocate to these feeding stations in search of free food, water, and medicine. If they stay, these farmers will then be away from their fields when the rains return the next season and will not be in a position to plant a new crop. They will become permanently dependent on food aid. Dislocations of this kind need to be avoided as long as food-stressed populations are still "coping."

Fortunately, a wide range of coping strategies are usually available in impoverished countries when temporary food shortages loom, including eating fewer meals every day, switching to less desirable "famine foods" (including wild foods that can be foraged or hunted in the bush), and selling off some farm animals or some nonessential household assets, such as jewelry, to raise the money needed to purchase food. Only when people run out of such options and begin taking more drastic steps, such as selling off essential farm implements, should they be encouraged to relocate to feeding camps, and even then they should be kept in this dependent condition only as long as necessary. Once the rains return or once the violent conflict ends, internally displaced persons should return to their farming communities. This can be encouraged by replacing the food aid with a one-time distribution of farm implements, animals, and cash—the things that people will need to return to a productive livelihood.

Can famine be prevented?

Famines are now prevented on a regular basis. In Africa, even large-scale drought no longer must result in famine. After a series of traumatizing emergencies in the 1970s and 1980s, the international community fortunately set in place for Africa a famine early warning system (FEWS) based on regular assessments of local rainfall patterns and market prices to ensure a more effective response to drought emergencies.

This system, operated by the FAO and the US Agency for International Development, proved to be highly effective in giving advance warning of food aid needs when drought struck southern Africa in 1991–1992. In Malawi, Namibia, Swaziland, and Zimbabwe, cereal production had fallen 60–70 percent, and 17–20 million people were placed at starvation risk throughout the region. Yet, thanks to an effective food assistance response from the UN World Food Programme (WFP), working in cooperation with local governments and humanitarian relief non-governmental organizations, the only famine deaths reported were in Mozambique, where aid was impossible to deliver because of an ongoing civil war. This new international capacity to prevent famine in Africa was then successfully tested a second time in southern Africa in 2001–2002, when drought returned and 15 million people were put at starvation risk. Once again, the international food aid response was timely, and essentially no famine deaths occurred.

Our modern international famine-prevention capacities can falter, however, in countries torn by internal conflict. In 2011 the Horn of Africa experienced its worst recorded drought in 60 years, and millions were placed at risk in Ethiopia, Kenya, Djibouti, and Somalia. The international community responded with a vigorous famine prevention effort, operated once again by the WFP. Famine was avoided everywhere except southern Somalia, where 50,000–100,000 people died. Famine deaths occurred there because southern Somalia was under the control of al-Shabaab, an armed jihadist militia group loyal to al-Qaeda that refused to let food aid come in. Famine dangers returned to Somalia late in 2022, with al-Shabaab still a threat, following four failed rainy seasons in a row plus a weak initial international food aid response.

5

INTERNATIONAL FOOD AID AND AGRICULTURAL DEVELOPMENT ASSISTANCE

What is international food aid?

Food aid is the international shipment of food through "concessional" channels as a gift, rather than through commercial channels, as a sale. The food can be given by a donor government to a recipient government, by a donor government to a non-governmental organization (NGO) working inside the recipient country, or through a multilateral organization such as the World Food Programme (WFP) of the UN. The food can be sourced from government-owned surplus supplies, purchased by the government in the donor country's home market, purchased from a local market in the recipient country, or purchased in a third-country market then shipped to the recipient country. The purpose of the food aid can be to address a temporary famine emergency (as described in the previous chapter), to cushion higher food prices (e.g., during the 2008 food price spike), to feed a dependent refugee population, or to support local work or education activities (through "food for work" programs, or school lunch programs). Food aid can generate cash income for development assistance organizations through sales into a local market (a process called monetization), it can dispose of a surplus, and in some cases it can be used to reward recipient governments for taking foreign policy actions pleasing to the donor government. Because there are so many ways to give food aid and so many different reasons for giving it, generalizations about this policy instrument are almost always dangerous.

One generalization can be made, however: food aid is less important to the world food system today than it was in the past. The assistance value of international food aid was $4.2 billion in 2020, with $2.5 billion of that coming just from the United States. This is a substantial amount, but as a share of all cross-border food shipments, food aid is now only 3 percent of the total, whereas in the early 1970s, it still made up about 10 percent of all cross-border food flows. The food aid share has decreased mostly due to a large expansion in commercial sales.

When has international food aid been important?

In the early 1950s, important food aid shipments came from the United States to support reconstruction in Europe following the damage of World War II, for example through the Marshall Plan. By the 1960s, the direction of most food aid had shifted toward South Asia, especially India, where food aid helped India avoid a famine, as mentioned in the previous chapter. Then, in the 1970s and 1980s, a great deal of American food aid went first to Vietnam and then to the Middle East, largely in service of foreign policy objectives. Finally, by the 1990s, Sub-Saharan Africa had emerged as the target destination of most food aid. According to one UN Food and Agriculture Organization (FAO) report in the 1990s, concessional international food aid provided more than 40 percent of total cereal imports for more than 40 recipient countries, and most of those countries were in Africa. In 2021, more than two-thirds of US food aid went to Sub-Saharan Africa, while another 20 percent went to the Middle East, where multiple refugee feeding requirements had emerged due to civil wars and armed conflicts. Wheat and wheat products make up the largest total tonnage of US food aid.

Food aid today moves less through bilateral government-to-government channels and more often through the UN World Food Programme. This change took place after an important UN World Food Conference in 1974, partly in response to the international food price crisis of that decade. By 2000, roughly 38 percent of all global food aid was delivered through the WFP, and by 2009, 64 percent of food aid was delivered through such multilateral channels. National governments in rich countries still fund nearly all food aid, but more than 90 percent of this aid is now distributed either by the WFP or by NGOs, rather than from government agencies.

The enlarged role of the WFP, a politically neutral UN agency, has helped to diminish the role of diplomatic favoritism in determining who gets aid and who does not. Unfortunately, this has made it easier for some recipient countries to become comfortable depending on food aid. In the 1960s, when most food aid came straight from the US government, often with diplomatic and foreign policy strings attached, recipient countries such as India became uncomfortable with the relationship and, partly to escape a dependence on food aid, made larger investments in their own agricultural production. Governments in Africa today that depend on food aid have shown less urgency in reducing their dependence because the food comes to them from the UN without any political conditions.

Do rich countries give food aid to dispose of their surplus production?

This was true for the United States in the 1950s, when domestic farm price support policies had generated a surplus quantity of wheat, which the government had to buy from farmers. One way to get this surplus out of government storage bins was international food aid. Under Public Law 480, enacted in 1954, also known as the Food for Peace program, government-owned surplus commodities could be shipped directly to recipient governments in the developing world. By 1960, fully 70 percent of US wheat exports were moving abroad as concessional food aid rather than commercial sales.

Later in the 1960s, however, the United States began supporting the income of its farmers with cash payments rather than through purchases of grain, so the amount of surplus food owned by the government dwindled. This might have brought an end to surplus disposal food aid, but by then it had become a convenient tool in the conduct of American foreign policy, so P.L. 480 did not disappear. Government-owned grain surpluses were gone by the 1970s, but Congress authorized the continuation of the food aid program based on government purchases of food in the marketplace, as long as it was purchased in the United States and then shipped abroad in US vessels.

How have America's food aid policies recently changed?

America's total international food assistance spending has roughly doubled since 2011, first in response to the larger needs that grew out of military conflicts in Syria, South Sudan, Somalia, and Ethiopia, and then as an emergency response in 2020 to the COVID-19 pandemic. The methods of giving food aid have also changed. Traditionally, nearly all US food aid was given "in kind," in the form of US grown commodities. Then in 2016 Congress passed the Global Food Security Act, which made it possible in emergency contexts to give cash for the purchase of food, including foods not grown on American farms. This kind of market-based assistance increased from 10 percent of total food aid outlays in 2011 to 57 percent by 2020. Most other major food aid donors, including Canada, the UK, and the European Union (EU), had already converted to giving assistance in cash rather than in kind.

This change made it possible to purchase and deliver food at a lower cost and with fewer delays in an emergency, but it was not universally popular. When President Barack Obama first called for changes of this kind in 2013, more than 60 domestic organizations, led by farm lobby and maritime lobby groups, signed a letter of objection to Congress. Farm lobbies wanted the food to be purchased only from American farmers, and the maritime lobby did not want to weaken requirements that 50 percent of the gross tonnage of American food aid be shipped on US-flag vessels (which are 70 to 80 percent more costly per ton than foreign-flag carriers).

Another controversial feature of American food aid has been the practice of selling the food into local markets rather than targeting deliveries more narrowly to needy recipients. Selling into local markets lowers food costs for the well-to-do as well as for the poor and hungry, and by undercutting market prices it can also disadvantage local farmers, thus prolonging dependence on food aid. This practice has persisted because some of the American NGOs handling the food rely on the monetary proceeds from local market sales to fund their other development projects. A number of leading American NGOs, including CARE, Oxfam America, Catholic Relief Services, and Save the Children, have signed a declaration, along with British, French, and Canadian aid groups, calling this practice into question.

Does food aid create dependence or hurt farmers in recipient countries?

In the early days of food aid in the 1950s and 1960s, when large shipments of surplus grain first went to the developing world as food aid, critics warned that a costly and dangerous dependence might result. Local consumers would become hooked on cheap food delivered from abroad, and local farmers would go out of business due to depressed food prices in the marketplace. Some even suspected that this was the American farm lobby's intent. Once the recipients had been lured into a dependence on food aid, the aid would be taken away and they would be forced to graduate to the status of paying customers.

Some American agricultural lobby groups may have hoped food aid would work in this manner as commercial export promotion, but it seldom has. America's largest food aid shipments in the past went to countries like Peru, Haiti, India, Indonesia, Vietnam, Jordan, Egypt, and the Philippines, and none of these later became a leading commercial market for US agricultural sales. By some estimates, more than half of all food aid actually displaced purchased shipments, meaning it destroyed more commercial sales in the short run than it ever created in the long run. Some of the commercial sales displaced were from other exporting countries, so food aid also triggered contentious trade disputes with rivals. When commercial sales do increase in the long run, it is usually because of income growth in the recipient country leading to more food demand. This means foreign investment and development assistance are actually far better tools for commercial export promotion than food aid.

There are some examples of food aid altering the behavior of consumers and food producers in recipient countries. Large deliveries of wheat and rice into West Africa in the 1970s accelerated local shifts in consumer demand away from sorghum and millet toward breads made from wheat. Large deliveries of maize as food aid to the Horn of Africa likewise encouraged recipients, many of them pastoralists, to shift their diet from animal products to grains. In most recipient countries, however, the quantity of food aid delivered has not been large enough inside the local market to trigger significant shifts in consumer behavior. Displaced communities who get food aid at refugee camps sometimes develop a dangerous dependence on the handouts, but entire national populations do not.

As a subsidy to domestic farmers in the United States, food aid also has limited impacts today because the shipments are so small relative to commercial agricultural exports and to the total cash sales made by farms. In 2019, the US government spent roughly $4 billion purchasing food aid, and only some of that food came from American farms; by comparison, total commercial agricultural exports from the United States that year were valued at $141 billion, and total cash sales by farms were close to $500 billion. Some individual commodity groups such as wheat and rice growers still count food aid shipments as a valued share of total sales, but for American agriculture as a whole the importance has become minimal.

Do governments use food aid to gain foreign policy leverage?

Governments have at times in the past been tempted to seek a coercive advantage by manipulating, or threatening to manipulate, the volume and timing of food aid shipments. During one prominent episode lasting from 1965 to 1968, President Lyndon Johnson did this to India by conditioning the continued delivery of food aid on changes that he wanted to see in Indian agricultural policy, and he also sought reduced Indian criticism of America's war policies in Vietnam. India had suffered two sequential harvest failures in 1965 and 1966 and was heavily dependent on deliveries of wheat assistance from the United States. Some of the agricultural policy changes that Johnson asked for were made, and most were good for India in the end, but India deeply resented the coercion and refused to end its criticism of American policies in Vietnam. The final political outcome was intensified Indian hostility toward the United States rather than compliant subservience.

Efforts to gain diplomatic leverage by manipulating commercial food exports are even more prone to fail. In 1980, President Jimmy Carter attempted to punish the Soviet Union for its invasion of Afghanistan with a partial embargo on US commercial grain exports, mostly wheat and corn. Carter's hope was that reduced imports would oblige the Soviets to cut back on the feeding of grain to cattle and pigs, resulting in meat shortages that might then reduce internal support for the Communist regime. The US embargo failed when other grain-exporting countries—particularly Argentina, Australia, and Canada—agreed to increase their exports to the Soviets to make up for the US sales being blocked. The Soviets, by offering only small price premiums to these other suppliers, were able to import roughly the same total quantity of grain during the US embargo as they had imported before the embargo. They meanwhile made the most of the embargo by blaming some of the meat shortages they were going to experience anyway on Jimmy Carter.

Food is hard to withhold for coercive purposes in part because most governments do not want to be blamed for imposing humanitarian hardships on foreign populations. In negotiations with North Korea over the distribution of American food aid, to make sure it would reach hungry populations, the United States paradoxically found itself at a disadvantage because any interruption of food aid could be depicted by North Korea as an American effort to use starvation as a tool of foreign policy, an accusation the United States wanted to avoid.

How is agricultural development assistance different from food aid?

Sending free food to countries in need is a valuable life-saving step in short-run circumstances, but the recipient countries would do better in the long run to make better use of the food production potential of their own farmers. Most farmers in poor countries are producing far below their potential, leaving many trapped in poverty and at risk of poor nutrition. According to the World Bank, average cereal yields in Sub-Saharan Africa in 2020 were only 1.5 tons per hectare, versus 3.4 tons in South Asia, 4.7 tons in Latin America and the Caribbean, 5.2 tons in East Asia, 5.4 tons in the EU, and 7.2 tons in North America. If governments in Africa gave farmers better access to improved seeds and fertilizers, better training through schooling and extension services, and better rural infrastructures for transport, storage, water, and electrical power, the productivity of farms would improve and the region's dependence on imported foods could quickly be ended. Agricultural development assistance is a form of "foreign aid" to help poor countries bring these vital assets to their own farmers.

Agricultural development assistance has been difficult for politicians in rich countries to support because it does not produce instantly visible benefits. Advocates for food aid, by contrast, can show photographs of refugee children whose lives are being saved by food deliveries. Most agricultural development programs, such as investments in agricultural research or agricultural education, do not deliver their full payoff for a decade or more, and attributing the benefit to the assistance will be difficult even then. Nonetheless, America's agricultural development assistance program, named Feed the Future, estimates that since it began operations in 2010, 23.4 million more people in the countries where it operates now live above the poverty line, 3.4 million more children are living free from stunting, and 5.2 million more families are no longer suffering from hunger. International assistance to support agricultural research delivers particularly strong benefits. The World Bank's *World Development Report 2008* documented rates of return on agricultural research in Africa that averaged 35 percent per year, accompanied by significant reductions in poverty. IFPRI has also estimated 50 percent average rates of return when the spending goes through Africa's own national agricultural research systems (NARS).

Investments in rural infrastructure also have large payoffs in the long run. In India, according to calculations done by IFPRI, investments in rural roads were even more powerful than investments in agricultural research for the purpose of lifting people out of poverty. Similar impacts have been measured in Africa. One IFPRI study in 2004 found that spending on rural farm to market feeder roads in Uganda had better than a 7 to 1 ratio of benefits (in terms of agricultural growth and rural poverty reduction) relative to costs. Supporters of agricultural development assistance believe that rich countries should use their foreign assistance programs to help poor countries make investments of this kind in rural infrastructure and agricultural research.

How much international assistance do rich countries provide for agricultural development?

According to the Organisation for Economic Co-operation and Development (OECD) headquartered in Paris, the world's rich countries provided a combined $12.6 billion in official development assistance to the agriculture, forestry, and fishing sectors of developing countries in 2020. This represented only 7 percent of all official development assistance, a relatively low percentage but one that has remained steady for a decade.

Two-thirds of agricultural development assistance moves through bilateral channels, and one-third through multilateral channels such as the World Bank, the EU, and the International Fund for Agricultural Development (IFAD). The largest share of this assistance goes to Sub-Saharan Africa, and the second largest share to South Asia. Almost one-third of the aid went for direct efforts to boost agricultural production, 15 percent went to support changes in agricultural policies, and smaller amounts went for agricultural education and research, rural development, and agricultural water resources.

Prior to the international food price spike of 2008 (discussed in Chapter 3), international assistance to agriculture had been in significant decline. In real terms, it had fallen 30 percent below the mid-1980s level. Following the price spike, a new political effort was made by development assistance advocates to return spending to the earlier levels, and these efforts paid off at a G8 meeting in L'Aquila, Italy, in July 2009, when President Obama persuaded rich country leaders to collectively pledge $22 billion for agricultural development over the next three years, of which $6 billion was to be new money. The president leveraged his argument by making a highly personal reference to the impoverished conditions still experienced by his own extended family living in the agricultural countryside in Kenya.

Many donor countries fell short of fulfilling this 2009 pledge. As the three-year period was coming to a close, a respected humanitarian NGO named the One Campaign reported that only about half of the pledged money had been disbursed or firmly committed. Even so, agricultural development assistance spending did increase markedly. In the United States, for example, annual congressional funding for bilateral and multilateral agricultural development assistance increased from $245 million in fiscal year 2008, up to $639 million in fiscal year 2009, and then all the way up to $1.3 billion by fiscal year 2012.

Much of this increase in US funding was then sustained when Congress enacted the Global Food Security Act of 2016, a bipartisan measure that formalized the status of President Obama's newly created Feed the Future program inside the US Agency for International Development (USAID). This program of assistance has been helping smallholder farmers since 2011 to make an additional $13.7 billion in new agricultural product sales, boosting their income.

Which agencies operate US agricultural development assistance?

Most US assistance programs for agricultural development are planned by officials from USAID and contractors for USAID working in coordination with individual recipient country governments. They are then largely implemented by non-governmental organizations from the United States, such as CARE or ACDI/VOCA. The activities funded in this manner include technical support and training for local farmer organizations, support for local seed and fertilizer dealers, and assistance in the marketing and processing of agricultural goods. USAID has significantly increased its own in-house capacity to design agricultural projects since the Obama administration launched its Feed the Future initiative in 2010, but most of the work on the ground continues to be outsourced to private contractors.

The other federal government agency that designs and funds significant agricultural development assistance programs is the Millennium Challenge Corporation (MCC), created by the George W. Bush administration in 2004 to provide an alternative to the USAID approach. The MCC operates by making bilateral five-year grants based on detailed "compacts" negotiated with recipient governments, which spell out the investments that will be made by the receiving government through its own locally established Millennium Development Authority (MiDA). Congress appropriates the full value of the compact before the agreement is signed, then the funds are disbursed by the MCC in installments. In the agricultural area, the MCC has specialized in funding infrastructure investments, such as an irrigation project in drought-prone Mali and rural road building in northern Ghana. Originally envisioned as a $5 billion per year program, the MCC has never been given adequate resources. Congress was not comfortable appropriating foreign assistance money five years in advance, and many Democrats have not been eager to support what was originally seen as a Republican innovation in assistance administration.

The United States also supports agricultural development through appropriations for the multilateral International Development Association (IDA) within the World Bank, plus a new Global Agriculture and Food Security Program (GAFSP), a pooled fund also managed by the World Bank. The GAFSP was created following a 2009 G20 Summit meeting, as yet another response to the 2008 food price spike. Unfortunately, international support for GAFSP proved weak, and even the United States faltered in supporting this fund, partly because the 2010 midterm elections put the House of Representatives into the hands of spending-conscious Republicans.

Who benefits from agricultural development assistance?

The beneficiaries include small as well as large farmers. In Ethiopia, for example, USAID has supported a Pastoralist Livelihoods Initiative that organizes women into groups to get credits that they can use either to buy sheep and goats or to diversify into horticulture production, and also a Productive Safety Net Program (PSNP) that funds local community-designed projects to build or repair rural roads, dig wells, plant tree seedlings, or construct school classrooms. These projects have paid off. When a record drought struck the Horn of Africa in 2011, Ethiopia avoided famine, and the number of citizens needing emergency food relief was only half as great as during an earlier drought in 2002–2003.

Increased agricultural development assistance to Bangladesh has also brought tangible benefits. Annual US assistance to Bangladesh grew from only $6 million in 2009 to $77 million by 2012. These funds made possible a number of initiatives, such as expanded use of a "fertilizer deep placement" technique that allows rice farmers to increase yields by 25 percent while reducing fertilizer use and runoff by 40 percent. The number of rural households benefiting directly from US agricultural development programs in Bangladesh increased from 119,000 in 2008 to 2,700,000 by 2012.

Does China also provide agricultural development assistance?

Since 2000, China has emerged as a prominent provider of development loans in the developing world, under its Belt and Road Initiative. According to China's Foreign Ministry, this global initiative has handed out roughly $1 trillion in loans to national governments in almost 150 different countries. The loans are politically directed by China's various state-owned financial institutions.

As one part of this larger effort, China began funding more ambitious agricultural development assistance lending in

Africa specifically. In 2000 it hosted a Forum on China-Africa Cooperation (FOCAC) in Beijing, and then began creating Agricultural Technology Demonstration Centers in individual African countries, of which there are now 25 in all. These centers often work through local universities, usually in association with Chinese companies, cities, and provinces. The activities of these Centers, along with various other Chinese agricultural investments in Africa, were valued at $13 billion by 2010.

When extending these loans, China's purpose is not just to improve the welfare of Africa's smallholder farmers. A deeper goal is to develop stronger political ties to African governments and to stimulate the production of agricultural goods that China itself may need to import in the years ahead, such as poultry from Kenya, sugar from Mozambique, or cotton from Mali, Uganda, and Zambia. For their part, African governments appreciate the fact that China's assistance projects—unlike USAID projects—are not conditioned on inconvenient requirements like democracy promotion, environmental protection, or human rights. China has also been willing to support large infrastructure investments in roads and irrigation, which are currently out of favor on environmental grounds with many Western donor governments.

The long-term impacts of China's agricultural assistance efforts in Africa remain an open question, in part because they have left some borrowing countries with debts that are hard to service, and also because Africa's smallholder farmers are frequently left in just a marginal role. The Chinese like to do everything themselves: they lease the land, then bring in expat workers from China to build out facilities and provide financial and technical support. The projects can perform well as long as the Chinese are in control, but when they go home things may fall apart. Earlier Western assistance efforts in Africa suffered from similar limitations.

6

THE GREEN
REVOLUTION CONTROVERSY

What was the green revolution?

The original green revolution, which took place in the 1960s and 1970s, was an introduction of newly developed wheat and rice seeds into Latin America and into the irrigated farming lands of South Asia and Southeast Asia. These new seed varieties had been developed by plant breeders working in Mexico and the Philippines with support from the non-profit Rockefeller Foundation. The new seeds were capable of producing much higher yields per acre if grown with adequate applications of water and fertilizer. By cross-breeding different seed varieties from all over the world, the plant scientists had managed to incorporate dwarfing genes that produced shorter rice and wheat plants that devoted more of their energy to producing grain, and less to straw or leaf material. Short, stiff straws also helped to hold a heavier weight of grain. The new green revolution seeds predated genetic engineering, so they were not GMOs. In fact, they were not even hybrid seeds. They had been developed through conventional cross-breeding, so unlike hybrids they kept all of their desirable traits when the seeds were saved from a harvest and replanted.

Farmers in India began planting the new wheat varieties in 1964, and by 1970 production had nearly doubled. The seeds were introduced not by private companies, but instead by nonprofit organizations such as the Rockefeller and Ford foundations, with support from donor agencies such as the US Agency for International Development (USAID) plus the government of India itself, which by the early 1970s was devoting more than 20 percent of its budget to agricultural development. Between 1964 and 2008, according to the UN Food and Agriculture Organization (FAO), average wheat yields per acre in India increased fourfold. New rice seeds gave an equally spectacular performance. In India, rice production in the states of Punjab and Haryana doubled between 1971 and 1976. In Asia overall, rice output had been increasing at only a 2.1 percent annual rate during the two decades before the new varieties were introduced in 1965, but output then grew for the next two decades at a much higher 2.9 percent rate. This significant boost in Asia's capacity to produce basic grains arrived at a critical moment when population growth was at its peak, and supporters of the new seeds credit this green revolution with saving the region from a dangerous food crisis. In 1970, the American scientist who did the most to develop and promote the new wheat varieties, Norman Borlaug, was awarded a Nobel Peace Prize.

Green revolution seed improvements did not end with wheat and rice. Significantly improved varieties of sorghum, millet, barley, and cassava had also been developed by the 1980s. Overall, more than 8,000 new seed varieties were introduced for at least 11 different crops. Robert Evenson, an economist at Yale University, calculated in 2003 that if these modern varieties had not been introduced after 1965, annual crop production in the developing world in the year 2000 would have been 16–19 percent lower than it actually was, and world food and feed prices would have been 35–65 percent higher.

Why is the green revolution controversial?

Despite offering dramatic production gains, the new seeds of the green revolution were surrounded by political controversy.

Some critics feared that they would lead to greater income inequality if only larger farmers were able to adopt them. Others worried that they would make farmers too dependent on the purchase of expensive inputs such as fertilizer. Still others feared environmental damage from excessive fertilizer applications, excessive pumping of groundwater for irrigation, or the excessive spraying of pesticides. The new seeds were also criticized on the grounds that they could reduce biodiversity if extensive monocultures of newly introduced green revolution varieties replaced diverse plantings of traditional crop varieties. Some critics even went so far as to argue that the green revolution seeds became a source of violent conflict in India, between Hindus and Muslims in the Punjab. In Central America, others blamed green revolution farming for rural dispossession and revolutionary violence.

Despite the controversies, the response of most farmers was to adopt the new seeds as quickly as possible, to secure the increased productivity and higher income. The most vocal critics of the green revolution were not farmers, but instead activists and political leaders who expressed faith in traditional practices, or who were suspicious of private seed and fertilizer companies, or who feared that coaxing higher yields from the land would prove environmentally damaging and unsustainable. The most outspoken green revolution critics, including Indian activist Vandana Shiva, called for a rejection of the new seeds, saying they would require more water and chemical use and reduce biological diversity.

These different views toward the original green revolution repeatedly resurface in contemporary political debates about food and farming. Supporters of the original green revolution encounter new resistance when they promote an extension of improved seeds, fertilizers, and irrigation to regions such as Sub-Saharan Africa. The original green revolution had little impact in Africa, due to a lack of road and water infrastructure and also because wheat and rice were not leading food staples in Africa. To overcome these barriers, the Rockefeller

Foundation and the Bill and Melinda Gates Foundation formed a partnership in 2006 called an "Alliance for a Green Revolution in Africa," or AGRA. Green revolution critics responded immediately that such a project would be a serious mistake. Peter Rosset, speaking for an NGO in the United States named Food First, warned that the most likely result of this new initiative would be "higher profits for the seed and fertilizer industries, negligible impacts on total food production and a worsening exclusion and marginalization in the countryside."

One explanation for these divergent views of the green revolution was the differing impact that the new seeds had in Asia versus Latin America. In Asia the benefits of the new seed varieties were widely shared by the poor, while in many parts of Latin America they were not. Today's advocates for the green revolution draw most of their evidence from the positive Asian experience, while critics like to reference the malfunctions they saw in Latin America.

Did the green revolution end hunger?

The green revolution helped reduce the prevalence of hunger in Asia today, compared to the hunger we would see if there had been no green revolution. Food became more abundant in the marketplace, and hence less costly for the poor, enabling increased consumption. It also boosted the productivity of farms and hence the incomes of the farmers who adopted the new seeds. It also benefited hired farm laborers, who found more work when harvests grew in size, as well as those who worked in the rural industries that thrived around the transport, storage, and processing of the additional food. These broad-based income gains brought improved nutrition. Studies done at the microlevel during the early years of the green revolution in Asia found that the higher crop yields typically led to greater calorie and protein intake among rural households within adopting regions. For example, economists Per Pinstrup-Andersen and Mauricio Jaramillo, examining the significant dietary improvements seen in one district in southern India in the 1980s, calculated that one-third of the increased calorie intake could be attributed to the increased rice production made possible by the new seeds.

The improved seed technologies of the Asian green revolution also triggered more rapid urban industrial development. In India, every 1 percent increase in the agricultural growth rate stimulated a 0.5 percent addition to the growth rate of industrial output, boosting incomes and reducing hunger in urban areas. China had a similar experience. When the government of China undertook reforms in 1978 that gave peasant households an incentive to make use of improved seed and fertilizer systems, agricultural production increased over the next two decades at an accelerated 5.1 percent annual rate, according to World Bank calculations, setting a foundation for the rapid urban industrial growth that soon followed. As a result, and despite continued population growth, the number of Chinese people unable to feed, clothe, or adequately house themselves declined from 250 million in 1978 down to 34 million by 1999, according to a 2000 development forum in Beijing.

Never before had so many people escaped poverty and malnutrition in such a short period. The uptake of more productive farm technologies had been key to this success; between 1975 and 1990, according to economists Jikun Huang and Scott Rozelle, the new rice technologies developed independently by Chinese researchers, such as hybrid rice seeds and single-season varieties, made possible over half of the yield increases behind the achievement.

Still, the green revolution by itself did not end hunger in Asia. Overall calorie consumption increased, but in some cases dietary diversity decreased as rice monoculture systems led to diminished consumption of leafy vegetables and fish. Elsewhere, the green revolution did not go far enough. In India, some rural communities were not touched by the green revolution due to inadequate rainfall and no irrigation, or because land tenure systems denied access to the poor. Economic growth rates increased in India overall, most dramatically after the 1990s, but in states such as Gujarat and Rajasthan there was limited improvement in nutrition, with persistent micronutrient deficits. In 2007, Prime Minister Manmohan Singh, in his 60th Anniversary Independence Day Address to the nation, candidly described India's malnutrition problem as "a matter of national shame." India today remains home to more than 40 percent of all the world's severely malnourished children.

Did the green revolution lead to greater rural inequality?

The answer is yes in Latin America, but not in most of Asia. Outcomes differed in these two regions because of some important underlying social differences in the countryside. In much of Latin America, ownership of productive land, and access to credit for the purchase of essential green revolution inputs like fertilizer, were restricted to a privileged rural elite. When a highly productive new farm technology is introduced into such a system, only the narrow elite will be able to take it up, so inequality will worsen. In most of Asia, by contrast, access to good agricultural land and credit was not so narrowly controlled, allowing the uptake of the new seeds to be more widely shared, with gains that were far more equitable.

Widespread social injustice continues to mark the history of farming in most of Latin America. Indigenous populations went into a tragic decline soon after Europeans arrived, falling an estimated 75 percent by 1650 due to a combination of brutal treatment by the Spanish and Portuguese conquerors plus a deadly exposure, with no acquired resistance, to unfamiliar European diseases. The Europeans then replaced indigenous farming systems with vast semi-feudal *hacienda* estates, on which peasants without land rights planted corn and beans on tiny plots for personal consumption while providing free labor for the landowner. To the present day, ownership of the best farming land in Latin America remains in the hands of a narrow rural elite. Poor peasants may own small plots of less productive land, but many own nothing at all. For every 100 smallholder farmers in Latin America who do own some land, 82 others do not.

These severe rural inequalities were in some places worsened by the introduction of green revolution technologies. The commercial farming elite adopted the new seeds quickly, partly because government subsidies were provided to help them purchase the fertilizers and pesticides used with the seeds. The top commercial farmers were also given subsidized credits, research and extension assistance, new irrigation canals for their fields, and exemptions from import duties on equipment like farm tractors, while poor farmers were excluded from these government benefits. Agricultural land was made more valuable by the new seeds, but this backfired on many poor farmers who had previously been allowed to plant corn and beans for subsistence on land they did not own. They would now be pushed off by the landlords, to make way for expanded commercial production of high-value crops like cotton. Some of the evicted peasants gained limited compensation in the form of seasonal employment as hired cotton pickers, but otherwise they were forced to shift their farming efforts onto more fragile sloping lands with no access to irrigation and with less fertile soil. Others decided to become slum dwellers on the fringes of the urban economy.

Asia had a different experience with the green revolution seeds, because so much of farming was dominated not by large estates but by smaller family plots, many with access to irrigation. Because the new seeds were a biological technology, it was not necessary to have a large farm to make use of them (the opposite is true for mechanical technologies, such as tractors). Even tenant farmers who rented land could use the seeds, so long as they had irrigation and could get access to credit to buy fertilizer. In fact, the International Rice Research Institute found, in one study of 30 rice-growing villages in Asia between 1966 and 1972, that small farms (less than 1 hectare in size) actually adopted the new seeds more quickly than larger farms (over 3 hectares in size). The higher-yielding green revolution varieties also increased farm labor demands, pushing up rural wages to the benefit of the landless poor. In some cases, inequality gaps developed between regions that had abundant irrigation and those that did not, but small as well as large growers benefited in places where farmers had water and credit.

The poverty reduction gains that came from the green revolution in Asia were dramatic. The International Food Policy Research Institute calculated that in 1975, early in the history of the green revolution, nearly 60 percent of Asians still lived on $1 a day or less. By 1995, this number had fallen to only 30 percent. Poverty continues to decline in rural Asia as improved farming technologies become pervasive.

Asian farmers both large and small have shown no interest in abandoning the green revolution, for obvious reasons. The critics warned that the early yield gains from the new seeds would not be sustainable, but yields have continued to increase. Data from FAO show that wheat yields in India in 2014 were 244 percent higher than when the seeds were first introduced in 1965, and rice yields were 177 percent higher. Yet the sustained technical success did not silence the critics. In 2004, a coalition of 670 separate NGOs sent an open letter to the director general of FAO referring to the green revolution as a "tragedy."

Was the green revolution bad for the environment?

The environmental impacts of the green revolution also differed in Latin America compared to Asia. In Latin America, two distinct kinds of environmental damage from green revolution farming often emerged side by side. On the best lands controlled by politically favored elites, government subsidies led to excessive irrigation, too much fertilizer use, and excessive sprays of chemical pesticides, creating occupational hazards on the farm plus pollution of the air and water downstream. In Mexico between 1961 and 1989, fertilizer subsidies led to an 800 percent increase in nitrogen fertilizer use per acre; over the decade of the 1970s, pesticide use increased at an average annual rate of more than 8 percent. In the Culiacan Valley, subsidized commercial tomato growers began spraying pesticides on their crops as often as 25 to 50 times each growing season.

Meanwhile, a different kind of environmental damage was done by poor farmers in Latin America who lacked subsidies and credits and did not participate in the green revolution. These farmers continued using too little fertilizer rather than too much, which exhausted their soils, forcing them to move onto even more fragile lands or into forest margins. In Honduras, where the population doubled between 1970 and 1990 and where the poorest two-thirds of all farmers were trapped on just 10 percent of the nation's total farming area, destitute peasants exhausted and eroded their soils, then cut much of the remaining forest cover. In Mexico, where half of all farmers were trying to subsist on only 10 percent of the nation's farmland, population growth among the rural poor led to an expansion of low-yield farming that devastated the environment. In the Mixteca region, according to a 1990 study by environmental scholar Angus Wright, 70 percent of the potentially arable land had lost its ability to grow crops due to soil erosion. Large parts of rural Mexico came to resemble a lifeless moonscape.

Excessive water and pesticide use became a problem in many Asian countries as well, due to unwise government subsidies, just as in Latin America. For example, in Punjab in northwest India in the 1980s, the government rewarded politically powerful commercial farming interests by paying 86 percent of their electric bill for pumping irrigation water. This resulted in excess water use and a precipitous drop in groundwater tables. In Indonesia in the early 1980s, the government subsidized fertilizer purchases by 68 percent, causing fertilizer use to grow by more than two-thirds. This increased nitrates in drinking water and brought nutrient runoff to streams and ponds, resulting in unwanted algae growth. Indonesia also offered an 85 percent subsidy to farmers who purchased pesticides, so excessive spraying on rice fields soon killed the good species, such as spiders, that had earlier helped to keep bad insects under control. The bad insects, such as brown planthoppers, in the meantime evolved to resist the chemical sprays. This finally prompted the government in 1986 to ban the spraying of 57 different insecticides on rice, a move that allowed the natural enemies of the hoppers to recover, eventually bringing the damage under control.

As serious as such green revolution problems were in Asia, the only thing worse for the environment might have been to introduce no high-yield seeds at all. If India had been forced to rely on its pre–green revolution, low-yield farming techniques to secure the production gains it needed during these decades of rapid population growth, there would have been no option but to expand the area under cultivation by cutting more trees, destroying more wildlife habitat, and plowing up more fragile sloping or dryland soils. According to M. S. Swaminathan, one of the scientists who led the green revolution in India, the new seeds helped India avoid "a tremendous onslaught on fragile lands and forest margins." In 1964, Swaminathan points out, India produced 12 million tons of wheat on 14 million hectares of land. Thirty years later, thanks to the green revolution, India was producing 57 million tons of wheat on 24 million hectares of land. To produce this much wheat using the old seeds would have required roughly 60 million hectares, implying that an additional 36 million hectares would have been put under the plow.

The charge that green revolution seeds require the use of more water and chemicals is widespread but technically mistaken. The use of these inputs did increase with the green revolution, but the new seeds produced so much more wheat and rice that the use of both water and fertilizer *per ton of production* actually declined. For fertilizer, the green revolution seeds produced more than 20 pounds of added grain for each added pound of nitrogen, while the traditional rice and wheat varieties produced only 10, so the need for fertilizer fell roughly in half for each pound of grain produced. For water use, FAO confirmed that the green revolution rice varieties actually increased water productivity threefold compared to traditional varieties, allowing only one-third as much water use for every ton produced.

Why did the original green revolution not reach Africa?

Green revolution farming has been slow to reach Sub-Saharan Africa. Between 1970 and 1998, while the share of cropped area planted to modern green revolution varieties increased to 82 percent in the developing regions of Asia, and up to 52 percent in Latin America, only 27 percent of such areas were planted to new varieties in Sub-Saharan Africa. As a result, crop yields remained unusually low in Africa. In 2020, according to the World Bank, average cereal yields in Sub-Saharan Africa were only 1.5 tons per hectare, versus 3.4 tons in South Asia and 4.7 tons in Latin America. Because of Africa's rapid population growth, these low yields have spelled trouble. FAO data show that Africa's cereal production per capita actually declined by 5 percent between 1980 and 2000. With so little gain in yield, Africa's only way to increase production has been to plow up more land, an environmentally damaging approach. Between 1980 and 2018, agricultural land use in Sub-Saharan Africa more than doubled.

Early efforts were made in the 1960s and 1970s to introduce green revolution seed varieties into Africa, but there was little adoption because the international assistance agencies introducing the seeds had tried to jump over the tedious and time-consuming step of breeding for yield improvements using locally adapted crops. Varieties not suited to African conditions were brought in from Latin America and Asia, and African farmers did not like them. This error was belatedly corrected when more location-specific breeding programs were launched at the beginning of the 1980s, but by then international assistance for such programs was declining. The success of the green revolution in Asia in the 1960s and 1970s, plus lower international food prices, had convinced many donors that the "world food problem" had already been solved, so they redirected funding away from agriculture, just at a moment when Africa was finally in a position to benefit.

African farmers were also slow to take up new seed varieties because their lands were ecologically more complex and often poorly suited to uniform, centralized systems. Access to farmland in Africa is generally more equitable than in either Latin America or Asia, but only 7 percent of agricultural land in Sub-Saharan Africa is irrigated. When farmers must rely entirely on uncertain rainfall, the incentive to invest in improved farming technologies weakens, since the investment can be wasted if the rains fail. Africa's weak rural road systems, which cut farmers off from markets, are another problem. Roughly 70 percent of rural Africans live more than 2 kilometers from the nearest all-weather road, making it hard to bring in fertilizers and seeds. Finally, Africa's dominant food crops were not wheat and rice, the crops that led the green revolution, but instead root crops like sweet potato or cassava, or other legumes and grains such as cowpea, white maize, sorghum, and millet.

More recently, improved farming technologies have begun to find their way into rural Africa, especially where there have been reductions in violent conflict, advances in democracy, and the growth of stronger civil societies. Government investments in agriculture have continued to lag, however. While India was devoting more than 20 percent of its public budget to agriculture early in its green revolution in the 1970s, most African governments have continued to spend less than 5 percent, despite having made public promises to spend twice that amount.

The 2006 AGRA initiative, plus increased efforts by international donors following the 2008 food price spike, led to modest increases in crop yields in some countries. In AGRA's thirteen participating countries, maize yields increased 29 percent over the first dozen years of the program. AGRA's $500 million in grants made over this period, mostly funded by the Bill and Melinda Gates Foundation, were focused more on seed improvements and seed systems than on building rural infrastructure. Recent data from the World Bank show that Africa's agricultural GDP growth rate increased from an average of 2.5 percent per year in the 1990s, which was no more than the rate of growth of population, to an average of 3.7 percent per year after 2007. Farm labor was being made more productive. Value added per worker in the farming, fishing, and forestry sectors had not increased at all in Sub-Saharan Africa between 1991 and 2001, but over the next two decades it increased by 72 percent.

What farming approaches do green revolution critics favor?

Critics of the green revolution believe that rural poverty can be reduced and farm productivity enhanced without introducing high-yielding seeds and more chemical fertilizers. These critics prefer farming models based on "agroecology," seen as an application of ecological principles to food production. This approach prefers farming systems that imitate nature, rather than those that try to dominate nature. This can mean using crop rotations and manuring rather than chemical fertilizers to replace soil nutrients, natural biological controls for pests rather than chemical controls, and mixing animals with crops. Polycultures (a variety of crops in the same field) are favored over monocultures, water-harvesting systems rather than large-scale irrigation, and a reliance on local community-based knowledge rather than laboratory science. Many advocates for agroecology start with a view that nature knows best. Human efforts to dominate biological systems will always fail, and can trigger unintended consequences.

One early advocate for agroecology as an alternative to the green revolution was Miguel Altieri, an ecosystem biologist originally from Chile, who looked at farming systems in Latin America in the 1980s, where the green revolution came in for early criticism. Altieri promoted an enhancement of traditional systems based on indigenous knowledge as an alternative to the foreign and reductionist green revolution approach. Altieri insisted on balancing any search for short-term productivity with an insistence on long-term stability, social equity, and sustainability. Green revolution advocates will contend that their approach can also be stable, equitable, and sustainable, as long as access to land and credit is widely shared, and as long as continuing investments are made in new seed varieties to stay ahead of evolving pest and disease pressures. Agroecology advocates mistrust this technical fix approach, doubting the ability of laboratory science to stay ahead of such pressures forever.

Advocates for agroecology have gained prominent endorsements for their views, and the approach has now won wide official support inside the UN system. In 2010, the UN Special Rapporteur on the Right to Food, Olivier De Schutter, described agroecology as the best way to guarantee the human right to food, and in 2013 the UN Conference on Trade and Development also endorsed agroecology. FAO convened its first International Symposium on agroecology in 2014, then it held a second symposium in 2018 where 700 government participants plus 300 non-state actors launched a new "Scaling Up Agroecology Initiative."

Scaling up agroecology will be difficult because farmers themselves usually resist. Agroecological methods, which often resemble hand gardening, are labor-intensive. Time must be spent building and repairing raised planting beds, pruning trees, carrying in mulch, recycling animal waste, and harvesting intercropped fields by hand. Such methods can work at the project level, when plenty of hired labor is available, but in their own fields and on their own time farmers tend to favor labor-saving green revolution methods.

Claims have been made for the success of agroecology in the country of Cuba, which had to abandon the heavy use of fertilizer when the Soviet Union collapsed after 1989 and Moscow stopped providing cheap chemicals. Agroecology advocates have said this led to improved outcomes but FAO data tell a different story. After three decades of experimenting with agroecology, Cuba's food production per capita has remained more than one-third below the level of 1990, and in 2019 Cuba had to introduce rationing of chicken, eggs, rice, and beans.

Fortunately, environmental concerns from farming can be addressed in the developing world without abandoning the gains of the green revolution. In 1997, Gordon Conway published a book calling for a "Doubly Green Revolution" that would combine animal manure with synthetic fertilizer use, and employ biological controls along with synthetic pesticides. Conway believed in using all the technical tools available for food production, so long as fertilizers and pesticides were used with restraint and precision. A more recent version of this integrated approach is Sustainable Agricultural Intensification (SAI), originally promoted by Jules Pretty, a biologist and professor of environment and society at the University of Essex. SAI does not insist on imitating nature, but it protects nature by reducing plowing, by using greater precision when adding inputs, and by using the resulting yield gains to minimize land use.

Advocates for agroecology accuse Conway and Pretty of proposing something that looks too much like "business as usual," yet their inclusive approach has the virtue of being more acceptable to farmers. The integrated methods they propose are something farmers can actually agree to adopt. In 2018 Pretty published an estimate that various SAI techniques— including integrated pest management (IPM), micro-irrigation, and reduced tillage farming—were already in use on 453 million acres around the world, or about 9 percent of agricultural land worldwide, so these are methods that can scale.

The most successful farming systems have always been those that integrate some agroecological techniques with green revolution seeds and other inputs. Crop rotations, such as planting a field with corn in one year and with soybeans in the next, are widely embraced by conventional farmers. Pest management techniques that integrate biological controls with chemical controls are another example. Combining agroecological techniques such as planting leguminous trees alongside a field of high-yield hybrid maize, then using a judicious amount of chemical fertilizer, is another integrated strategy.

One rapidly growing system for integrating agroecology with conventional farming has been "no-till" farming, in which farmers do not plow the ground before planting. Instead, they use specialized machinery to sow seeds directly through crop residues from the previous harvest. This method retains soil moisture, protects the soil against erosion from runoff, sequesters carbon in the soil, and saves time and money by eliminating plowing. Conventional farmers in the United States started moving toward this method in the 1970s, originally as a response to high fuel costs, and now the technique has spread to many other countries as well. In 2012, IFPRI reported that on the Indo-Gangetic Plains, Indian farmers using reduced tillage practices spent an average of $55 per hectare less in cultivation costs, saved 50–60 liters of fuel and 15–50 percent of water, and increased their crop yields by 247 kilograms per hectare. Methods such as these can help put the green revolution on a more sustainable path.

How have green revolution critics shaped international policy?

The political controversy over green revolution farming versus agroecology continues to rage, particularly within the UN system where environmental and social justice NGOs have gained a strong voice. These NGOs continue fighting to promote agroecological and organic approaches to farming, in place of green revolution methods, and this advocacy did begin to have an impact on the foreign assistance policies of donor countries in the 1980s. International assistance was cut back for new irrigation projects in the developing world, new seed development, and sales of chemical fertilizers.

Between 1980 and 2003, the real dollar value of all bilateral assistance to help modernize agriculture in the developing world declined by 64 percent, from $5.3 billion (in constant 1999 US dollars) to just $1.9 billion. US assistance to new agricultural research in Africa declined by 77 percent. This withdrawal of donor support had little effect in Latin America and Asia, where agricultural modernization had already taken off and become self-sustaining, but it left aid-dependent governments in Africa without enough external support to begin a confident move of their own down the green revolution path.

Even with revived concerns about the world food supply following the international food price spike of 2007–2008, the green revolution approach remained under a political cloud. The new concerns did lead to increased donor assistance for agricultural development, particularly in Africa, but always against background warnings from critics that the green revolution path would sooner or later prove unsustainable. Green revolution critics even argued that the higher international food prices were, in some way, proof that the gains from current methods had been exhausted. Actual measures of total factor productivity growth in conventional agriculture did not support this view. A 2008 study by economist Keith Fuglie in the journal *Agricultural Economics* revealed that, among the developing countries as a whole, the growth rate of total factor productivity in agriculture had been twice as high in the 1991–2006 period as during the earlier 1970–1990 period.

Green revolution critics have continued to push back. In 2021, when a UN Food Systems Summit was convened in New York, more than 500 NGOs boycotted the event in part because the secretary-general had named a Rwandan agricultural scientist, Dr. Agnes Kalibata, to be his special envoy to the summit. Kalibata was president of the Alliance for a Green Revolution in Africa, an initiative seen by NGOs as corporate-led and incompatible with agroecology.

The green revolution continues to be criticized by most organized environmentalists and social justice advocates in rich countries, yet it remains the approach of choice among most farmers and agricultural policy leaders in the developing world. In China and India today, green revolution seed varieties grown in monocultures with nitrogen fertilizer remain the dominant production model, continue to be strongly supported by the state, and have brought continued productivity gains.

7

THE POLITICS OF OBESITY

Is the world facing an obesity crisis?

Worldwide, obesity rates have roughly doubled in the last four decades. In 1980, 5 percent of men and 8 percent of women around the world were obese. By 2016, the rates had increased to 11 percent for men and 15 percent for women. According to the World Health Organization (WHO), most of the world's people now live in countries where obesity and overweight cause more deaths than hunger and underweight.

Obesity prevalence in the United States has increased even more. In 1964, America's obesity rate for adults was 13.4 percent and increasing only slowly. In the mid-1970s this rate began a more rapid rise, and by 2010 it reached 36 percent, and then 42 percent in 2018. Other wealthy societies are experiencing increased obesity as well, and urban populations in middle-income countries have also joined this global trend. One 2020 study predicted that as many as 1.5 billion people around the world will be obese by 2050, roughly twice the number who are undernourished today. The world has been slowly winning its battle against undernutrition, but it now faces a new and increasingly pervasive challenge from over-nutrition.

How do we measure obesity?

Obesity is a crude measure of the roundness of the body, based on a body mass index (BMI): body weight (in kilograms) divided by the square of height (in meters). People with a BMI between 25 and 30 are considered overweight; those with a BMI above 30 are obese; and those with a BMI above 40 are described as severely obese. Translating to more familiar terms, a six-foot-tall individual is considered overweight above 183 pounds, obese above 220 pounds, and severely obese above 295 pounds. Adverse health consequences are far more likely when individuals go from merely overweight to obese. Those in the United States who are moderately obese have personal health care costs 20–30 percent higher than those with a healthy weight, while severe obesity more than doubles health care costs. Some studies show that obesity, on average, reduces life expectancy by six to seven years.

Between 1971 and 2018 in the United States, the prevalence of obesity among adults roughly tripled, going from 14.5 percent to 42 percent. Between 2000 and 2018, the rate of severe obesity among adults increased from 3.9 percent to 9.2 percent. In other words, nearly 20 million adult Americans are now 100 pounds or more above what is considered a healthy weight. Among children ages 6–11 in the United States, the rate of obesity has increased even more rapidly, from 5 percent in 1980 up to 20 percent by 2018. In 2012, the Robert Wood Johnson Foundation projected that if obesity rates continued on the current trajectory, 39 states will have rates above 50 percent by 2030, and all 50 states will have rates above 44 percent.

America leads other rich countries in the prevalence of obesity, but many others are following a parallel path. In Canada, 26.8 percent of adults were obese in 2018. In Mexico, one 2022 study found that 30.5 percent of adult men were obese, and 40.2 percent of adult women. Even in Japan, which has one of the lowest obesity rates in the world (6.7 percent for men,

3.9 percent for women), obesity rates for men in their 20s have doubled over the past three decades.

What are the consequences of increasing obesity?

Obesity has become a serious medical problem in America, helping to bring on a growing burden of chronic disease, especially type 2 diabetes, cardiovascular disease, and cancer. The National Institutes of Health estimates that obesity may be linked to 300,000 deaths per year in the United States.

Obesity is technically defined as a physical condition, not a medical condition; it is perfectly possible for individuals to be both heavy and healthy. According to Dr. Robert Lustig, an expert on childhood obesity, 20 percent of obese people have completely normal metabolic signatures, and conversely up to 40 percent of normal-weight people have the exact same metabolic problems that the obese do, even though they are not obese. Even for diabetes, BMI alone cannot be blamed, since this illness can be linked to sugar consumption independent of body weight. Nonetheless, in 2013 the American Medical Association voted to categorize obesity itself as a "multi-metabolic and hormonal disease state," a move that might open the way for obese citizens to seek larger benefits from the government for treatments and accommodations.

As obesity rates have gone up in the United States, the medical community (including organizations like the American Heart Association and the Academy of Nutrition and Dietetics) has sought increased measures for prevention, but most Americans have found it easier to focus on treatment and accommodation. This is not an unusual response in America. One 2020 study found that more than a quarter of medical spending in the United States goes for the treatment of diseases that could have been prevented. There is an Obesity Action Coalition that lobbies Congress for more pharmaceutical treatments such as weight-loss drugs, while the American Society of Metabolic and Bariatric Physicians pushes for surgical treatments. Surgical treatments for obesity carry high cost and significant risk, but for those in greatest need, particularly those who are severely obese, surgical procedures such as "gastric bypass" can bring both permanent health gains and also reductions in long-term medical costs.

Obesity is primarily a personal and a family concern, but the compounding medical costs have made it a public health issue as well. In the United States between 1998 and 2008, the medical costs of treating obesity-related diseases doubled to reach $147 billion, or about 9 percent of all medical costs. Compared with someone of normal weight, medical spending for a person with obesity is 42 percent higher per year. By 2030, if trends continue unchecked, obesity-related medical costs could rise by another $48–$66 billion a year in the United States.

Some of the largest costs of obesity can be personal, in the form of reduced employment and income options, social isolation, and depression, but days missed from work, more frequent hospitalizations, and more expensive medical insurance have social as well as personal impacts. Obesity is even a national security issue. In 2010, a panel of retired military officers found that 27 percent of all young adults in America were "too fat to serve in the military." Between 1995 and 2008, the percentage of potential recruits who failed their physicals due to being overweight increased by nearly 70 percent.

What is the cause of today's obesity crisis?

Obesity results when the human body persistently takes in, through eating and drinking, more caloric energy than it burns through basic metabolism and muscular exertion. The modern obesity epidemic derives from both an increase in average caloric intake and a decrease in average muscular exertion. Person by person, genetic inheritance helps explain some of the occurrence of obesity within generations, but it cannot explain the rapid increase we have seen in prevalence across generations, because human genetics does not change that fast. A breakdown in personal discipline also cannot explain this rapid increase. The obesity rate in America has tripled since 1970, and it simply can't be possible that Americans today are three times as irresponsible as they were back then.

Increased calorie intake is the single largest source of the problem. In the United States between 1970 and 2003, average daily caloric intake increased 23 percent to a level of 2,757 calories, which was roughly 20 percent more than the World Health Organization recommends. Meanwhile, average muscular exertion declined, as people walked less and drove more, and as physical demands in both the home and the workplace were reduced. Most work in America now takes place while sitting in chairs, or behind the wheel of a vehicle. In the home, the physical work of cleaning rugs, dishes, and clothing is now done with electrical power rather than muscular exertion. Snow removal, grass cutting, and hedge trimming have all been motorized. Washing automobiles is now automated, and seasonal chores such as hanging storm windows no longer exist. Stair climbing has been replaced by elevators. Only 8 percent of middle schools and 2 percent of high schools now require daily physical education for all students. While 20 percent of trips between school and home were on foot in 1977, that figure had fallen to just 12 percent by 2001.

Despite a booming fitness industry, working out has actually declined. Among American men 40 to 74 years of age, since 1990 the number of people who report exercising three times a week has dropped from 57 percent to 43 percent. Only 23 percent of American adults meet leisure-time physical activity (LTPA) guidelines, according to a 2018 study from the Centers for Disease Control (CDC). Even before the COVID-19 pandemic, more leisure time was spent sitting in front of home computers, television, or smartphones. The average American adult now spends about 6.5 hours a day sitting, up about an hour a day since 2007. For teenagers ages 12 to 19, that number is eight hours a day.

Does cheap food cause obesity?

Personal calorie consumption in America has increased in part because food has become cheap, especially relative to income. Over the course of the 20th century, the real cost of food commodities declined by 50 percent in the United States, thanks primarily to productivity growth on the farm, while average consumer income was at the same time increasing by roughly 400 percent. Food today is so cheap relative to income that increasing quantities are wasted and simply thrown away. The average American wastes more than 700 calories of food per day, and between 2010 and 2016 the amount of food wasted in the United States increased by 12 percent.

The low cost of food in America is sometimes blamed on farm subsidies. One leading advocate for this view is journalist Michael Pollan, who told one university audience in 2017, "[W]e create incentives for our farmers to grow huge quantities of corn and soy, mostly in the Midwest. Corn and soy is really where the calories in most of the junk food come from . . . we have inadvertently created a system where the cheapest calories in the supermarket are the least healthy."

Most agricultural economists disagree with this explanation. Farm support policies throughout the industrial world tend to make food artificially expensive, not artificially cheap, largely because they include restrictions on imported foods, including foods that worsen obesity like sugar. This is even more the case for Europe and Japan than for the United States, but significant sugar import restrictions in the United States nonetheless make all sweeteners more expensive, not cheaper. One study by three economists published in the journal *Food Policy* in 2008 found that if national farm subsidy policies were eliminated in the United States, the cost to consumers of sugar, soybeans, rice, fruits and vegetables, beef, pork, and milk would go down. A later study published in *Health Economics* in 2012 showed that if all farm subsidies were removed—including the measures that reduce imports of cheap food from abroad—the cost to Americans of sugar and dairy products would be even lower, inducing a further increase in calorie consumption for a typical adult.

Critics often assert that farm subsidies in the United States have generated too much corn production, which in turn lowers the price of livestock feed, making meat products artificially cheap. To the contrary, corn prices are currently being propped up due to federal policies, especially the government mandates that require the use of corn for ethanol production, which reduces the quantity left over for food and animal feed. The price of corn has also been driven up by import restrictions on sugar that encourage the use of corn-based sweeteners, such as high-fructose corn syrup (HFCS). If sugar import restrictions were removed, the price of both sugar and HFCS in the United States would fall, making sodas, candy, and ice cream even cheaper, and the obesity crisis would worsen.

In one respect, US policies do make food artificially cheap for low-income households, through nutrition assistance programs like the Supplemental Nutrition Assistance Program (SNAP), but obesity has been increasing among citizens who don't qualify for SNAP benefits, so this also fails as a promising overall explanation.

Another charge, that junk food prices have fallen in the United States while fruit and vegetable prices have not, is also questionable. A 2008 study by the Economic Research Service at the US Department of Agriculture (USDA) showed that over the previous 25 years the price of fruit and vegetable products in the marketplace (controlling for quality and season of the year) fell at almost exactly the same rate as the price of chocolate chip cookies, cola, ice cream, and potato chips. Not only are fresh fruits and vegetables cheaper than ever before when sold in season, they are also more widely available out of season.

Unhealthy snack foods are on average no cheaper than healthy snacks. When USDA compared dollar costs, it found that for 20 healthy fruit and vegetable snacks the average cost per portion was 2 cents lower than for 20 food snacks that were less nutritious.

Healthy foods are also more available in American supermarkets than ever before. Over a single decade in the 1990s, the average number of produce items in America's supermarkets doubled. Between 1970 and 2014 the per capita availability of fresh fruit increased 40 percent, even after adjusting for spoilage, plate waste, and other losses along the supply chain. The total availability of fresh vegetables per capita increased 21 percent. The per capita availability of broccoli, specifically, increased 14-fold.

Do fast foods and junk foods cause obesity?

Yes, but other foods are a problem as well. In 2011 the *New England Journal of Medicine* published a study revealing that the top contributors to weight gain in the United States included red meat and processed meats, sugar-sweetened beverages, and potatoes, including mashed potatoes and French fries. The single biggest weight-inducing food was the potato chip. Other studies suggest that the single largest driver of the obesity epidemic has been sugar-sweetened beverages (SSBs). In one study of overweight and obese high schoolers, when the sugary drinks normally consumed were replaced with sugar-free alternatives, average weight loss over a 12-month period was 4 pounds. Fortunately, consumption of these beverages, including juices, dairy drinks, sports drinks, and sweetened soft drinks, peaked in 2000 at 263 calories a day and has been in significant decline on a per capita basis, down to 198 calories a day by 2017.

Consumption frequency and meal portion size also explain part of America's obesity crisis. In the 1970s, children in the United States consumed an average of just a single daily snack, but by 2012 three daily snacks was the average, adding almost 200 daily calories to the diet. Meanwhile, average entrée portions from fast food chains in the United States delivered 90 more calories by 2016, compared to 1986. Nutrition policy expert Marion Nestle said in a 2014 interview: "Large portions are a sufficient explanation for why people are gaining weight. It's not because of lack of exercise; it's because we're eating more."

It is sometimes alleged that the sweetening of beverages with high-fructose corn syrup rather than natural sugar has made these drinks more obesity inducing, but the evidence to support this charge is weak. The HFCS used in soft drinks consists of 55 percent fructose and 45 percent glucose, not significantly different from ordinary sugar, which is 50 percent fructose and 50 percent glucose. Michael Jacobson, former director of the Center for Science and the Public Interest (CSPI), has said that the popular idea that HFCS carries a greater obesity risk is "an urban myth."

Fast food (or "quick service") restaurant meals have long been an invitation to more obesity. It is not unusual for an individual meal to contain more than 1,000 calories. It takes an hour and 20 minutes of jogging to burn off that much energy. Careful studies that control for variables such as income, education, and race have shown that obesity rates among ninth-grade schoolchildren are 5 percent higher if the school is located within one-tenth of a mile of a fast food outlet. Restaurant chains that serve sit-down meals are also part of the problem. A brief published in the *Journal of Nutrition Education and Behavior* in 2014 found from a study of 21 full-service chain menus in Philadelphia that the average meal—consisting of an adult entrée, side dish, and shared appetizer—delivered 1,495 calories (plus 28 grams of saturated fat, and 3,312 mg of sodium). If a nonalcoholic beverage and a shared dessert are added, the calorie total for a single meal goes above 2,000.

As the obesity crisis has worsened, restaurant chains have worked hard to include more "healthy choices" on their menus. In 2009, Burger King announced three new kids' meals that included smaller burgers, sliced apples designed to look like French fries, reduced-sodium chicken tenders, and fat-free chocolate milk. McDonald's began to offer apples and yogurt.

Taco Bell developed an entire menu of vegetarian options, and Pizza Hut reduced the sodium in its products. The Food Network now endorses 23 different fast food chains as healthy.

Are food companies to blame for the obesity crisis?

Yes, to a large extent. These companies do more than simply package and deliver foods to consumers. They also design and process food products and restaurant meals with an eye to making them virtually addictive, in part by adding sugar, salt, and fat. The added sugars give us calories we do not need, while leaving our appetite unsatisfied, so we are hungry again far too soon. Processed foods with carefully formulated tastes and textures are intentionally designed to hit a "bliss point," triggering the reward circuit in our brain, ensuring we will soon want to repeat the experience. In his 2021 book *Hooked*, Michael Moss compared the addictive quality of these scientifically designed food company products to cigarettes and cocaine. Food companies also ultra-process their products, leading to faster eating and still more consumption. One 2019 study found that eaters served exactly the same foods, but in an ultra-processed versus a minimally processed form, take in an average of 508 added calories a day.

Between 1994 and 2006, food companies in the United States introduced about 600 new children's food products; half were candies or chewing gums, and another one-fourth were other types of sweets or salty snacks. The companies advertise these foods to children who are not old enough to understand the health implications of consuming high-calorie, low-nutrient junk foods. The CSPI asserts that the food and beverage industry spends $2 billion every year advertising food to children. Kids aged 2–11 years see an average of 13 food ads a day. The companies go beyond television ads, also targeting children who use smartphones and laptops. One favorite vehicle has become free online games, available on sites like Candystand.com. On this site Kraft Foods released an iPad app, "Dinner, Not Art," in which players slide pieces of mac and cheese around the screen to create macaroni art.

The United States does less to regulate food advertising than most other wealthy countries. In 1980, Congress barred the Federal Trade Commission from making broad new rules on food advertising to children. Under pressure, some companies have at least taken voluntary action. In 2012, the Walt Disney Company announced it would no longer accept advertisements for junk food on its child-oriented television and radio sites. In 2022, the consumer packaged goods company Unilever announced it would stop advertising food and drink products to children under the age of 16.

As calorie consumption has increased overall, the consumption of many nutritious foods in America has actually declined. Federal guidelines recommend that adults eat at least 1.5 to 2 cups per day of fruit and 2 to 3 cups per day of vegetables, yet the CDC reported in 2015 that only 12 percent of adults met the daily requirement for fruit, and just 9 percent for vegetables. Multiple factors have driven such long-term trends, including more people working outside of the home (resulting in fewer home-prepared meals), more commuting by car and a rapidly growing preference for meals that can be held in one hand while driving, greater leisure time spent snacking while watching television, and also less cigarette smoking (an appetite suppressant).

Companies that sell packaged foods, represented by the Consumer Brands Association (CBA), which was formerly the Grocery Manufacturers Association (GMA), attempt to present themselves as guardians of consumer health and well-being, saying they are "committed to helping arrest and reverse the growth of obesity around the world." The responses to the obesity crisis they favor include "consumer education" and "personal responsibility," but not taxes or regulations. The companies claim they are only giving consumers what they want, and have been forced by market competition into selling foods with too much sugar, salt, and fat. According to Geoffrey

Bible, a former chairman of the board of Kraft Heinz, "If we give them less, they'll buy less, and the competitor will get our market. So you're sort of trapped." In such circumstances, governments should step in to reduce this damaging competition by setting common standards for all.

The pressure on food companies to do better has produced some results. Kraft Heinz itself has introduced a no-added-sugars version of Capri Sun juice, and Oscar Mayer hot dogs without byproducts, and even a mac-and-cheese product with no artificial coloring. Smuckers now has 22 different jam and jelly products that are reduced sugar or sugar-free. Frito-Lay has introduced healthier versions of its chips to limit sodium and saturated fat, while adding more fiber, whole grains, vegetables, and protein. In 2016, according to the Consumer Goods Forum, food companies improved the health profile of about 180,000 products, compared to just 80,000 in the previous year.

In 2005, the US Department of Health and Human Services jointly with the Department of Agriculture published new Dietary Guidelines for Americans, which recommended that half of daily grain intake should come from whole grains. In response, bread companies voluntarily reformulated products so they could claim a higher whole grain content (yet some then defeated the purpose by making the reformulation more palatable with added quantities of sugar, salt, or fat). In 2006, the Food and Drug Administration began to require disclosure of trans fat content on food labels, and New York City banned trans fats in restaurant foods. This experience induced a number of food manufacturers, including Nestlé, Kraft, Campbell's, Kellogg's, and Frito-Lay, to reformulate products to eliminate trans fats entirely, and several major food service companies, including McDonald's and Burger King, announced their intent to begin using frying oils with no trans fats. KFC began replacing trans fats before they had to, in anticipation of the New York City ban.

Supermarket chains have made efforts as well. Delhaize America has been promoting a system called Guiding Stars, which rates the nutritional value of most of the food and beverage products sold in their stores. Foods that have more vitamins, minerals, dietary fiber, and whole grains, and less fat, sugar, sodium, or cholesterol are given stars. Research suggests customer purchases in these supermarkets have shifted measurably toward the products that have been awarded stars. Yet the political power of the food industry has blocked any move to make such systems mandatory.

Do "food deserts" cause obesity?

Obesity is a growing problem for nearly all categories of Americans. Between 1994 and 2008, according to the Centers for Disease Control and Prevention, the prevalence of obesity increased in adults at all income and education levels. Yet factors such as residency, income, education, and race do make a difference. Some of the highest obesity rates are found among African Americans and Hispanics, especially women who live at lower income levels in underserved areas, including areas with a shortage of supermarkets selling fresh fruits and vegetables. Such areas, known as "food deserts," have been widely suspected as playing a role in the nation's crisis of unhealthy eating. Where there is a shortage of supermarkets selling fresh fruits and vegetables, residents may have no choice but to eat at fast food restaurants, or to purchase energy-dense packaged and processed foods from corner convenience stores. When the USDA examined this idea using data from the 2010 census, it found that almost 10 percent of the US population, or roughly 30 million Americans, did live in low-income areas more than 1 mile from a supermarket.

Under careful study, however, a convincing link between limited access to supermarkets and obesity has been difficult to establish. The best recent scholarship suggests that our eating habits have worsened not because our access to fresh fruits and vegetables has declined, but because we are now surrounded and tempted throughout the day by a pervasive presence of unhealthy ultra-processed food products, which are found not just in fast food restaurants and convenience stores, but also in gas stations, airports, and even pharmacies. We are not suffering from food deserts so much as we are drowning in food swamps.

One 2017 study defined a food swamp as a neighborhood with a high ratio of fast food restaurants and convenience stores to supermarkets and grocery stores. If a neighborhood had four unhealthy places to buy food for every one deemed healthy, it was classified as a swamp. By contrast, food deserts were mapped out based on the share of the population with both low income and low access to supermarkets or grocery stores. This study found that food swamps were stronger predictors of obesity than food deserts. In fact, the contribution of food deserts to obesity became statistically insignificant once you controlled for food swamps. Another study in 2021 found that "[t]here is so far little evidence that food deserts have a causal effect of meaningful magnitude on health and nutrition disparities."

Building more supermarkets in food deserts has not been a guaranteed solution in any case, because the center aisles of many supermarkets are actually a part of the swamp. Only 30 percent of the manufactured food products in supermarkets are good for health, according to a study funded by the Robert Wood Johnson Foundation.

Low-income households in the United States suffer from less favorable health outcomes across the board, and obesity is just one of those outcomes. For low-income households, having too little time for meal preparation can be almost as damaging as having too little income. A single working parent with young children may find it more convenient to pick up a bucket of KFC fried chicken on the way home, rather than shopping at a market for healthy foods that require more preparation and cleanup time.

Increasingly, our meals are not taken at home. Back in the late 1970s, only 17 percent of total average daily energy intake in the United States came from foods prepared away from the home, but by 2012 that had doubled to reach 34 percent, as the number of away-from-home food service establishments in the country had nearly doubled. Prior to the COVID-19 pandemic, Americans also were taking more meals while commuting to work: 17 percent of all meals ordered from restaurants in America were being eaten in cars.

Unstructured eating of this kind is no longer unique to the United States. Throughout Europe, a rapid increase in the number of women in the workforce has undercut traditional at-home meal preparation, leading to a parallel shift toward the consumption of high-calorie fast foods and convenience foods. In the United Kingdom, 27 percent of all food spending is now for meals from outside the home, and in Spain, 26 percent. Even in France, time spent on meal preparation at home has fallen by half since the 1960s. Fast food restaurants have been on the rise even in Greece and Portugal. The much-praised Mediterranean diet (based on vegetables, fruit, unrefined grains, olive oil, and fish) is now less prevalent even in Mediterranean countries. Nonetheless, obesity prevalence on the continent of Europe remains only half as high as in the United States.

What government actions are being taken to address the obesity crisis?

In the United States, strong government actions to reduce obesity—such as taxes on sugar-sweetened beverages—are favored by many advocates for public health, but most citizens object to such actions as "nanny state" infringements on their personal freedom. This strong resistance to government intrusion is a distinctly American attitude. In one 2011 Pew Global Attitudes survey, Americans preferred "freedom to pursue life's goals without state interference" over "state guarantees that nobody is in need" by a margin of 58 percent to 35 percent. In Britain this preference was roughly reversed, with only

38 percent preferring freedom. In Germany and France, 62 percent opted for state guarantees over freedom. Accordingly, governments in Europe, as well as in Asia and Latin America, have enjoyed more room to take strong actions to prevent obesity. The strongest policies are often found in countries like Japan where problems with obesity were never far advanced.

The US government also takes weak action on obesity prevention because most health care costs in America are still paid through employer-provided private health insurance systems, rather than through a shared tax burden. In addition, many in America claim not to see obesity as a problem at all. Close to half of all obese Americans say that their own body weight is not an issue, and more than 40 percent of parents with obese children describe their child as being "about the right weight." Social acceptance of obesity is actively promoted by civil rights advocates for the overweight, led in the United States by the National Association to Advance Fat Acceptance (NAAFA), an organization that has been operating since 1969.

Governments have a wide array of policy options to push back against obesity. At the least coercive end of the spectrum, they can try public education campaigns about healthy eating, require health ratings on packaged foods, or require calorie counts for restaurant meals. More coercive steps might include restrictions on advertising of some foods to children, or mandatory counseling by primary care physicians. Subsidy policies might be used to reduce the price or increase the availability of nutritious foods, and tax or regulatory policies might be used to increase the price and reduce the availability of energy-dense, non-nutritious foods. On the physical activity side, governments could move back to requiring physical education in schools, or invest more in playgrounds, bike paths, and sidewalks. Mandates, taxes, and regulations are normally the strongest policy instruments available to governments, yet one 2010 study by the OECD revealed that governments in wealthy democratic societies were primarily relying on weak policies like subsidies to increase the consumption of healthy foods, rather than strong measures like taxes or regulations to reduce unhealthy consumption.

One exception in the United States is a federal rule that came into effect in May 2018, requiring restaurants with 20 or more locations to post calorie counts on their menus and menu boards. The rule also applies to foods on display in supermarkets, convenience stores, and movie theaters, plus nearly all of the nation's 5–6 million vending machines. It took 15 years for Congress to pass this law, in the face of strong resistance from the restaurant industry. The overall benefit is still uncertain, but one review of calorie counts by the Cochrane Collaboration found that people did reduce calorie consumption, on average by 48 calories per meal, or about 8 percent.

A more typical political outcome in America has been the unwillingness of Congress to remove sugary beverages from the SNAP (food stamp) program. Supported by public health experts, this idea has consistently been rejected not only by the beverage industry, but also by the anti-hunger lobby, which does not want any restrictions at all on the items low-income households can purchase with SNAP benefits, making it easier for the beverage industry to prevail. To lock in the advantage, leading companies like PepsiCo and Coca-Cola give generous financial contributions to anti-hunger lobby groups like FRAC (the Food Research and Action Center).

A number of countries beyond the United States are now taking much stronger measures against obesity. Many have enacted "front-of-package" nutrition guidance schemes that give food shoppers, at a glance, clear information on potential health risks. The UK has a "stoplight" system that shows either green, yellow, or red lights to indicate whether the quantities per serving of things like sugar and salt are within safe limits. Government-endorsed systems of this kind are now also in place in Croatia, Czechia (the Czech Republic), Denmark, Finland, France, Iceland, Israel, Lithuania, Norway, Poland, Slovenia, Sweden, Belgium, and the Netherlands. Some of these systems consist of just a simple endorsement logo (a heart symbol, or a green keyhole) that signal at a glance the "healthier choice" foods.

America's currently required Nutrition Facts panel provides only small print and numbers, and it is on the side of the package rather than the front. Private food companies in America have developed their own voluntary "Facts Up Front" nutrition labeling system, but it lacks an "at a glance" feature. At the 2022 White House Conference on Hunger, Nutrition, and Health, President Biden announced that the FDA would study options for stronger front-of-package nutrition labeling, but this is a political minefield that timid FDA bureaucrats have shied away from in the past.

Many European countries also restrict the advertising to children of foods high in sugar, salt, or fat. Ireland prohibits the advertising of such foods during children's TV and radio programming, and it has overall limits for other times of day. The UK has a similar rule for viewers under 16. Norway prohibits ads on children's programs, plus marketing to children under 18. In France, all TV advertising for processed foods and drinks that contain added fats, sweeteners, or salt must be accompanied by messages such as, "For your health, avoid eating too many foods that are high in fat, sugar, or salt."

Restricting food ads to children has been politically impossible in the United States, since the Supreme Court ruled in 1976 that advertising was "commercial speech" protected under the First Amendment. The Obama administration tried to prepare voluntary federal guidelines for food ads to kids, but the top lobbyist for the Grocery Manufacturers Association condemned the proposed guidelines as a "dramatic overreach," and Congress in 2011 passed a measure killing the effort.

An even stronger policy measure is the taxation of unhealthy foods, especially sugar-sweetened beverages. Governments in the UK, France, Hungary, Catalonia, Mexico, Portugal, South Africa, Peru, and the Philippines have all done this, but in the United States consumption-reducing taxes on sugary beverages have never been enacted at either the state or federal level. Since 2014, however, a number of municipalities have taken this step, including Berkeley, Philadelphia, San Francisco, Oakland, Albany (California), Boulder, and Cook County, Illinois (which includes Chicago). The Cook County decision was later reversed, and a local tax effort failed in Santa Fe in May 2017, but Seattle joined cities opting for a soda tax the following month. These municipal tax measures could be undertaken thanks to three factors: strong Democratic Party control over city government; announced plans to dedicate the tax revenues to a specific purpose other than deficit reduction; and external financial support to promote the effort from private foundations, especially Bloomberg Philanthropies.

Municipal soda taxes can produce the intended result. Soda consumption was cut by one-fifth in Berkeley, and in Philadelphia soda sales fell by 38 percent in 2017, even when increased purchases in neighboring towns are taken into account. Purchases in Seattle dropped 30 percent in the months after the tax took effect. Results like these are the reason beverage industries fight back hard, and are working to preempt local taxes through state legislatures where their lobby is stronger. Extending municipal soda taxes to other cities, and eventually to the state and federal level as well, could lead to considerable improvements in dietary health.

The strongest national legislation currently in place against obesity in the United States is the 2010 Healthy, Hunger-Free Kids Act. This law reformed the National School Lunch Program, which provides meals to 31 million children a day. The new 2010 law expanded the number of low-income children eligible for meal subsidies, so long as schools served increased portions of fruits, vegetables, and whole grains, while limiting sodium, fat, and calories. Advocates for regulating school menus pointed to a 2007 initiative in Mississippi that led to a 13 percent decline in obesity among elementary school children. Doubters cautioned that students consumed only about

25 percent of their calories in school, weakening the reach of this policy instrument.

The 2010 law was also blunted when the frozen pizza industry secured language from Congress qualifying pizza (with tomato sauce) as a vegetable. Potato farmers then managed to block curbs on how often French fries could be served. The responses of schoolchildren to the 2010 law were also mixed, as vegetable servings often ended up in the trash. Nonetheless, one 2021 study found that since 2010 school meals had become among the healthiest meals American children will encounter on an average day.

A related federal initiative was First Lady Michelle Obama's 2009 "Let's Move" campaign to reduce childhood obesity. In addition to public education, this campaign sought to persuade Walmart, Walgreens, Supervalu, and other grocers to commit to locating more stores in low-income neighborhoods. In one response, a team of grocery industry groups, health care organizations, and banks committed $200 million to eliminating "food deserts" in California. As noted earlier, however, building more supermarkets remains an unproven strategy for reducing obesity.

Who lobbies for and against stronger policies on obesity?

In the United States, the most visible advocates for stronger policies to prevent obesity include public interest lobby groups such as the CSPI, private foundations dedicated to improving health such as the Robert Wood Johnson Foundation, and university-based think tanks such as the Rudd Center for Food Policy and Obesity at Yale University. Individuals who are obese and citizen groups with members who suffer from obesity are not usually in the lead. Those who suffer from obesity more often organize for social acceptance and accommodations, or for the purpose of seeking more affordable treatments. Taxes on sodas or energy-dense snack foods can easily be depicted as regressive, making them unpopular even within the low-income or minority communities where obesity is a serious problem. For example, the president of the National Association for the Advancement of Colored People openly opposed New York City mayor Michael Bloomberg's 2012 move to ban large servings of sugary drinks, and in 2010 when New York asked for permission to exempt soda from SNAP coverage, leaders from the minority community criticized the move as an insulting suggestion that SNAP recipients were not capable of making smart food choices. A 2013 survey from the Associated Press and the Center for Public Affairs Research revealed that 70 percent of Americans support requirements to post calorie counts on menus, and 80 percent would support requiring more physical activity in school, but 60 percent are opposed to taxes that target unhealthy foods. Only one-third considered obesity a community problem; most viewed it as an issue primarily for individuals.

The strongest opposition to more effective obesity policies in the United States comes from the food and beverage industry, which argues that what we decide to eat should be a personal choice. Kevin Keane, a spokesperson for the American Beverage Association, said in 2009, "It's overreaching when government uses the tax code to tell people what they can eat or drink." When the City of New York attempted to restrict the sale of large drinks in 2012, it was sued by the American Beverage Association, the National Restaurant Association, a soft drink workers' union, and groups representing interests ranging from movie theater owners to Korean American grocers. Nationally, a Center for Consumer Freedom, funded by the restaurant and food industry, regularly criticizes any government effort to shape or reduce food choices.

Weak obesity-prevention policies in the United States also derive, to some extent, from the social influence of groups organized not for obesity prevention but for treatment. Pharmaceutical and medical companies profit from selling treatments, not cures, for those who develop type 2 diabetes, high blood pressure, and high cholesterol. In contrast, many employers and insurers have a greater interest in prevention than in treatment. The United Health Group has offered a health insurance plan in which a $5,000 yearly deductible can be reduced to $1,000 if a person is not obese and does not smoke. Financial inducements have even been tried. In 2009, the National Health Service in the UK ran a pilot program that offered cash payments of up to 425 pounds sterling depending on how much weight was lost (the program was called "pounds for pounds"). Nearly 800 people joined the scheme, but most dropped out. Those who completed the program lost weight, but many subsequently gained it back.

From a public policy perspective, governments must take care not to view excessive calorie consumption as parallel to cigarette smoking, alcohol abuse, or narcotic drug use. Unlike tobacco, alcohol, or narcotics, calories from food are absolutely essential to human health. And unlike smoking, being obese poses no "passive" health risk to others. Social risks such as impaired driving, domestic violence, and criminal behavior are also missing in the case of obesity. Most important, a significant share of obese people are quite healthy, and for some individuals the condition is driven more by genetics than lifestyle. Government policies that punish or stigmatize such individuals must be avoided. The best intervention is usually private counseling from family members or a trusted personal physician.

8

THE POLITICS OF FARM SUBSIDIES AND TRADE

Do all governments give subsidies to farmers?

Nearly all governments in rich countries subsidize the income of farmers. In 2021, according to calculations by the Organisation for Economic Co-operation and Development (OECD), government policies in 38 rich countries boosted the income of farmers by a total of $245 billion, either through tax-funded subsidies or by propping up farm commodity prices. On average, 15.9 percent of total farm receipts in these countries came from such government policies, down from 30 percent in 2000. In some rich countries the subsidy share of farm income is much higher (49 percent in Norway, and 37 percent in Japan), and in others much lower (only 8 percent in Mexico). In the United States, 10 percent of farm receipts depended on government interventions in 2021, while in the EU it was 18 percent.

The policies that transfer this income to farmers include direct cash payments, market or trade restrictions to boost crop prices, subsidies to cheapen the purchase of crop insurance, and subsidies intended to reinforce environmentally sustainable planting practices. In the United States, most income transfers to farmers come at the expense of taxpayers, but in countries that support farm income primarily through import restrictions—such as Japan, Korea, Norway, and

Switzerland—most of the transfer comes at the expense of consumers, who are forced to pay higher prices for food. There is a popular belief that farm subsidies make food cheap for consumers by boosting production, but as previously noted, this is not the case. The purpose of farm subsidies is to boost the income of farmers, not to boost food production. Import restrictions do encourage added domestic crop production, but not enough to make up for the blocked imports, so the prices that domestic food consumers pay are still artificially high, not artificially low.

Governments in poor developing countries provide much less income support to farmers, despite the fact that farmers in these countries are more numerous and usually disadvantaged relative to urban dwellers. In fact, poor countries often impose policies that tax their farmers, while subsidizing food costs for urban consumers. In India, government policies in 2021 reduced the income of farmers by 8 percent, and policies in Argentina reduced farm income by 19 percent. These countries sometimes tax or block food exports, or they rig their internal markets to oblige farmers to sell food at an artificially low price, thus creating an income transfer away from farmers and toward food consumers. Farm and food policies in many poor countries thus tend to be urban-biased, while in rich countries they tend to be rural-biased.

What explains the tendency of all rich countries to subsidize farm income?

Governments usually start subsidizing farmers during the initial stages of their industrial development. All economic sectors gain income and wealth during this industrialization process, including the agricultural sector, but larger farms will start to buy up smaller farms, since a bigger size makes it easier to take advantage of newly available powered machinery such as tractors and harvesting combines. This mechanization process leads to an out-migration of labor from agriculture and hence to farm consolidations. Rural towns will begin to depopulate, small shops will struggle, and public schools will also have to consolidate or close. Confronting these socially difficult challenges, smaller farmers will usually organize to seek assistance or protection from government. Feeling they are losing out in the economic marketplace, they will form lobby groups to strengthen their voice in the political marketplace, demanding income support through tax breaks, subsidized loans, import restrictions, market interventions to raise crop prices, and even direct cash payments.

The countries of Europe were the first to industrialize, so they were also the first to provide subsidy programs of this kind to support farmers, initially during and after World War I. The United States began regulating agricultural markets and providing subsidy benefits to farmers a bit later, during the Great Depression of the 1930s, through the Agricultural Adjustment Act (AAA) of 1933, as part of President Franklin D. Roosevelt's New Deal program. Japan embraced agricultural subsidy policies even later, when that nation moved toward full industrial development in the 1950s and 1960s; in Taiwan and South Korea, subsidies came still later, when rapid industrial growth reached those countries in the 1970s and 1980s.

The magnitude and timing of this policy response to industrialization has been carefully examined by economists. One 1986 study, by economists Masayoshi Honma and Yujiro Hayami, of the protection offered to farm sectors across the industrial world, found that 60 to 70 percent of all variations in the protection level given to farmers could be explained solely through reference to the comparative economic advantage being lost by the agricultural sector relative to the industrial sector, which is essentially a measure of the industrial development transition.

Do farmers in rich countries need subsidies to survive?

When farm subsidies were initiated in the United States in 1933, most farmers were relatively poor, with average incomes less than half that of non-farmers. At this point, in the depths

of the Great Depression, income support for farmers had social and economic justification. This justification began to diminish, however, when millions of poor farmers left the land
during and after World War II, to take higher-paying jobs in
urban industry. The result was a consolidation of farms into
much larger and more productive units, most of which no
longer needed subsidies to prosper. Because of continuing
farm consolidations, the greatest share of all food production
in America today comes from very large commercial farmers,
with average family incomes significantly higher than the
non-farm average. The average income for all family farms
in America in 2016 was more than 40 percent above the average for non-farm households, and the average net worth of
farmers is higher still thanks to the valuable land, buildings,
and machinery they own.

There is no such thing as an average farm in America. The
nation has 2 million farms but most produce very little of our
food. More than four out of five are either retirement farms,
part-time farms, or farms with few sales. America's larger
farms—the 146,568 farms with annual sales above $500,000—
make 81 percent of all product sales, even though they represent just 7 percent of all farms. In 2017, the American Enterprise
Institute published a study advising Congress to terminate
many farm subsidy programs, since they sent too many tax-
payer dollars to these large, wealthy farms. This advice was
ignored in 2018, when Congress passed yet another farm bill
renewing these programs.

Large commercial farmers do not need subsidies to remain
prosperous, yet they continue to get the largest share of the
subsidies. Most farm subsidies remain linked to current or
past production volume, so the biggest farms get the biggest
subsidies. In the United States in recent years, 5 percent of all
farms have received 45 percent of all agricultural subsidies. The
same pattern prevails in Europe, where the wealthiest 20 percent of farmers typically receive over 80 percent of the subsidies.

Efforts to tighten the targeting of subsidy payments are
routinely blocked by lobbyists representing large commercial

farmers. In 2008, President George W. Bush proposed to Congress that the law should be changed to prevent the delivery of some subsidy payments to farmers who earned more than $200,000, but the Senate determined instead that the cap should instead be set higher at $750,000, and the House of Representatives said there should be no cap at all.

Why are farm subsidies hard to cut?

Non-farmers outnumber farmers by at least 20 to 1 in most rich countries, yet they seldom mount effective campaigns to cut farm subsidies. In part this is because city people respect the heritage of farming and want to help those working on the land, yet few have any idea how poorly targeted the subsidies are. In addition, because of the "logic of collective action" originally spelled out by economist Mancur Olson, smaller numbers of farmers will naturally find it easier to organize for political action than the much larger numbers of consumers and taxpayers. Very large groups (like food consumers) find it hard to organize because nonparticipation is harder to notice, and thus to discipline. For the same reason, some smaller commodity groups (e.g., sugar farmers) do better at getting subsidies than larger commodity groups, such as wheat or soybean farmers.

Also, as the total number of farmers continues to shrink with industrial development, the average benefit *per farmer* can continue going up without translating into a higher budget cost overall. Moreover, if the budget cost of farm support does increase in a wealthy country, it may scarcely be noticed alongside the rising costs of much larger budget items, such as health care costs, or defense spending. Finally, when farm supports make food more expensive in rich countries, increasingly affluent consumers may not notice because food spending will still be falling relative to their income. The average share of personal income spent on food in the United States has fallen from 41 percent a century ago to just 10 percent today. This drop would have been even greater without farm subsidies, but this is something consumers either don't know or don't notice.

Despite these powerful political forces that tend to keep subsidies in place, once the farming share of the national workforce shrinks to a small enough size (below about 5 percent), the level of support given to farmers will usually reach a peak and begin to decline. At this point, the number of farmers will become too small, and their prosperity too conspicuous, to sustain a continued growth in subsidy benefits. Popular concerns about the environmental impacts of large-scale "industrial" farming will also undercut support for farm subsidies. This has now happened in both Europe and the United States. Between 2000 and 2011, the amount of income transferred annually to farmers through government programs in Europe declined by 21 percent, and in the United States by 40 percent. In the EU in 2021, a new "Farm to Fork" environmental strategy under the "European Green Deal" was opposed by farm lobbies (the German Farmers' Association called it a "general attack on the whole of European agriculture"), but when it went before the European Parliament in October 2021 it won strong majority approval. Europe's farm lobbies were able to out-muscle Green Parties in the past, but now the shoe is on the other foot.

What is the "farm bill" and what is the "farm lobby"?

The legislative package that renews America's farm subsidy entitlement system roughly every five years is known as the "farm bill," and the organized groups that promote the subsidies provided by this bill are known as the "farm lobby." Passage of the farm bill is a process controlled almost entirely by Congress. President George W. Bush tried to veto the 2008 farm bill because it carried a five-year budget cost of $286 billion that he considered wasteful, but Congress easily overrode his veto, by margins of 316–108 votes in the House and 82–13 votes in the Senate.

The secret to every farm bill's success in Congress has been a lead role played by the Agricultural Committees of the House and the Senate, where members from farm states enjoy a dominating presence, and are rewarded for their efforts with generous campaign contributions from organizations representing the farmers who get the subsidies. The Agriculture Committees draft the legislation that later goes to the floor for a final vote, and in the drafting process they take care to satisfy the minimum needs of both Republican and Democratic members, ensuring bipartisan support within the committee. The farm bill enacted in 2002 actually passed the House Agriculture Committee without a single dissenting vote. The drafters give generous treatment both to Northern crops (such as wheat and corn) and Southern crops (such as cotton and rice). Then they add some measures to please environmentalists, such as a "Conservation Reserve" program that pays farmers to leave their land (temporarily) idle. Finally, they tie federal nutrition programs like SNAP (food stamps) to the bill, to lock in voting support on the floor from urban members. The final package becomes impossible to stop; it is what students of legislative behavior call a "committee-based logroll."

Once the farm bill leaves the committees and reaches the floor, classic vote trading provides a final push toward successful enactment: farm state members implicitly or explicitly promise that they will vote for future measures of interest to non-farm members. For urban and suburban members, a single "aye" vote on the farm bill once every five years thus pays off when their own pet projects later come up for a vote.

This farm subsidy renewal process is supported by a formidable nexus of institutions often referred to as an "iron triangle." At the congressional corner of the triangle are the House and Senate Agriculture Committees, populated and chaired by strong farm subsidy advocates. At the executive branch corner is the US Department of Agriculture (USDA), which administers not just the farm subsidy programs but also the nutrition programs like SNAP, which it guards as protection against diminished departmental relevance in a post-agricultural age.

At the third corner of the triangle are the private farm lobby organizations. The best known of these are two "general" farm organizations, the American Farm Bureau Federation (commonly known as the Farm Bureau), which represents the interests of large commercial farmers, mostly Republicans, and the National Farmers Union, which represents the interests of smaller farmers, mostly Democrats. When it comes to shaping the details of the farm bill, however, the most influential private lobby organizations are those representing individual commodity producer groups, such as the National Corn Growers Association, the US Wheat Associates, the National Cotton Council of America, or the National Milk Producers Federation. These organizations make contributions to the re-election campaigns of their favorite Agriculture Committee members and send their affable and well-informed operatives to work the member offices and halls of Congress during the committee drafting process.

The continuing clout of the farm lobby was particularly visible in the outcome of the 2008 farm bill debate, which took place at a time when most of America's farmers were enjoying enormous prosperity thanks to the highest market prices for farm commodities seen in more than three decades. Net farm income in 2008 reached $89 billion, 40 percent above the average of the previous 10 years. Yet the farm lobby asserted that American agriculture was facing "emergencies" of various kinds and needed a new "safety net" for protection. The 2008 bill thus included added spending for research on organic agriculture and specialty crops, new conservation measures, block grants to promote horticultural products, and a new Average Crop Revenue Election (ACRE) program.

The routine renewal of farm subsidies proved more difficult in 2012, and again in 2018, in part because of Republican concerns that the SNAP program had become too large, but in

December 2018 Congress nonetheless enacted a new $867 billion farm bill (over 10 years) by wide bipartisan margins: 386–47 in the House and 87–13 in the Senate. Political sympathy for commercial farmers was momentarily high due to damage felt by soybean producers and hog farmers from President Trump's trade war with China. These farmers also exercised their political influence outside of the farm bill process, by securing an additional $28 billion in direct payments from USDA's Commodity Credit Corporation in 2018–2019 as compensation for the export sales to China they had lost.

Is the use of corn for ethanol a subsidy to farmers?

Agricultural crops such as sugar or corn can be fermented to produce ethyl alcohol (ethanol), which is then blended with gasoline for use as an automobile fuel. Beginning in 1978, Congress began promoting the use of corn for fuel by providing tax credits to those that blended ethanol with gasoline, and by setting in place tariffs to block the import of cheaper sugar-based ethanol from Brazil and the Caribbean. The promotion of corn-based ethanol was subsequently ramped up under the Energy Independence and Security Act of 2007, when Congress added a mandate that ethanol use from products like corn should total at least 15 billion gallons by 2015. The ostensible purpose of this new Renewable Fuel Standard (RFS) was to reduce America's dependence on imported oil for reasons of national security, but there were also clear financial benefits to the ethanol industry and corn growers, both of which were strong advocates for these measures.

The new government mandate helped trigger a dramatic expansion of the ethanol industry in the United States, accompanied by an increasing diversion of corn into fuel production. Between 1983 and 2010, ethanol production jumped from 2.8 billion gallons to 13 billion gallons, and by 2012, the percentage of America's corn harvest processed in ethanol distilleries had reached an astonishing 40 percent (however, about one-third of what is processed returns to the agricultural market as high-protein feed for animals). Some of this diversion of agricultural crops to fuel use would have taken place even without government subsidies and mandates, given the higher market price for petroleum after 2005. When petroleum prices are high and corn prices are low, market forces alone will divert more corn into use as a feedstock for fuel. The subsidies and mandates accelerated the growth of a corn-based ethanol industry in the United States, but if the price of oil goes high enough, ethanol production will expand even without government props.

The 2007 law set high long-term targets for renewable fuel production (36 billion gallons by 2022) that have not been met. This is because the so-called second-generation cellulosic feed stocks, such as switchgrass and wood chips, proved too costly to scale up, while the use of more corn also became impossible because the US auto fleet was not equipped to use ethanol blends with gasoline higher than 10 percent. The advantage of cellulosic feed stocks would have been freeing up more corn for use as food and animal feed, bringing down food costs for consumers around the world, but the production costs have remained too high.

What is the value of promoting corn-based ethanol in the United States?

Corn-based ethanol can sometimes make commercial sense, but on energy security and environmental grounds it makes very little sense. In the search for national energy independence, ethanol from corn can never offer more than a small gain. According to one 2007 study in the journal *Regulation*, even if 100 percent of the US corn crop were processed for ethanol, the total share of national gasoline consumption displaced would be just 3.5 percent.

The environmental consequences of switching from fossil fuels to corn-based ethanol are also unappealing, in part because fossil fuels must be burned while planting, harvesting, and processing the corn, as well as to manufacture the required fertilizers. Growing more corn for use as fuel also has adverse land-use implications. A 2008 study by Joe Fargione in the journal *Science* concluded that when worldwide land-use changes are taken into account, the greenhouse gas emissions from first producing and then burning corn-based ethanol are greater than those from producing and burning gasoline. It makes greater environmental sense, and also greater commercial sense, to burn ethanol that has been produced from sugar rather than corn, yet policy in the United States promotes ethanol from corn, because corn is what American farms produce.

How do farm subsidies shape international agricultural trade?

The farm subsidies of rich countries have long distorted both production and trade. They cause too much food to be produced in regions not well suited to farming, such as alpine countries in Europe, or desert lands in the American Southwest, or municipal suburbs in Japan, and too little in the developing countries of the tropics where agricultural potential is often far greater. Farm subsidies in the United States, Europe, and Japan also tend to take market shares away from other rich countries more advantaged with farming assets, such as Australia or New Zealand. Sugar markets are one example. Because of the guarantees of high sugar prices still being provided through import restrictions in both Europe and the United States, too much of the world's sugar production comes from growing sugar beets inside these two markets rather than from sugarcane in the Caribbean, Brazil, or tropical Africa. D. Gale Johnson, a highly respected agricultural economist, once calculated that because of protectionist farm subsidy policies, at least 40 percent of the world's sugar crop was being grown in the wrong place.

When international commodity prices are moving downward, these distortions can worsen the hardships faced by

farmers in the developing world. In 2002, the Brazilian government raised a formal complaint against American cotton
subsidies, showing that without those subsidies production in
the United States would have been 29 percent lower, cotton
exports from the United States would have been 41 percent
lower, and international cotton prices for Brazilian growers
would have been 13 percent higher. This would have brought
benefits not only to Brazil but also to small cotton farmers
in West Africa, many of whom lived on less than $1 a day.
According to calculations commissioned by Oxfam America,
if United States cotton programs had been eliminated in 2005,
and if the international price of cotton had consequently
increased by 6–14 percent, eight very poor countries in West
Africa would have been able to earn an additional $191 million
in foreign exchange each year from their cotton exports, and
household income in these countries would have increased by
2.3 to 5.7 percent.

Has the WTO been able to discipline farm subsidies?

One purpose of the World Trade Organization (WTO) has
been to reduce trade distortions caused by farm subsidies,
and successive rounds of multilateral trade negotiations in the
WTO (and within its predecessor organization, the General
Agreement on Tariffs and Trade, or GATT) made some progress in the 1990s in achieving this goal. Agricultural tariffs
around the world remain substantially higher than tariffs for
manufactured goods, but they came down in the United States
to just 5 percent, in the EU to 12 percent, and in Japan to 16 percent. In many developing countries, however, tariffs on agricultural goods remain high, averaging 38 percent in India.

Barriers to international agricultural trade can be difficult
to bring down in some rich countries because domestic farm
support policies would be far more expensive for governments
to operate without them. In Europe and Japan, it is politically
easy to transfer income to farmers through trade restrictions

at the border because these do not cost anything in budget terms (they may actually earn tariff revenue for the government), and they push costs onto foreign producers who complain, but cannot vote. In poor countries, meanwhile, barriers to agricultural trade are hard to bring down because they frequently reflect a political desire for "self-sufficiency" in staple food supplies. Even when their own people are not well fed, and even when prices on the world market may be lower than the domestic price, governments in many developing countries have traditionally preferred not to import staple foods.

Within the WTO, a distinction emerged in the 1990s between subsidies to farmers that distort production (and hence trade) versus those that do not. One WTO strategy has been for governments to negotiate limits on trade-distorting subsidies only, while approving unlimited cash subsidies to farmers so long as those payments are "decoupled" from any incentive to produce more. Payments that supposedly do not incentivize new production are placed in a "Green Box," while policies that clearly distort production are placed either in a "Red Box" (they are banned) or in an "Amber Box" (where they are allowed, but only up to a certain dollar value). Following this approach in the Uruguay Round of WTO negotiations that ended in 1993, the United States and Europe were able to agree to reduce their Amber Box supports by 20 percent from a 1986 baseline. Following this agreement, both the United States and the EU voluntarily decoupled larger portions of their farm subsidy budgets, so they could be moved into the Green Box and increased without WTO restriction.

Even with this Green Box loophole in place (plus a second, more dubious loophole known as the Blue Box), it proved impossible after 2001 to reach a follow-up agricultural agreement in the next round of WTO negotiations. This Doha Round was suspended without a result in the summer of 2008. The talks failed when some developing countries—including both China and India—said no. They believed any new access they might gain to agricultural markets in the United States and the EU would not be enough to justify the new concessions they were being asked to make in opening their own domestic markets for both agricultural and manufacturing goods. Agreements in the WTO are reached on a "consensus" basis, which makes agreements more difficult to reach as the number of major economic powers has increased. The emergence of Brazil, India, and China as stronger economic powers after the 1990s made the task of reaching a multilateral consensus on agriculture in the WTO far more daunting.

Do trade agreements like NAFTA hurt farmers in countries like Mexico?

When global negotiations in the WTO falter or stall, the United States sometimes attempts to open markets abroad through regional or bilateral trade agreements. In his 2013 State of the Union address, President Obama signaled a desire to negotiate a Transatlantic Free-Trade Agreement (TAFTA), parallel to a possible Trans-Pacific Partnership (TPP) free trade agreement. Securing EU or Japanese support for these approaches would have required offering a "carve-out" provision to limit or exclude any further reductions in farm subsidies. Neither of these initiatives came to fruition, however, thanks to a broad political retreat from free trade enthusiasm in the United States, first driven by pro-labor Democrats fearing a further loss of industrial jobs, and then by populist "America first" pro-Trump Republicans who distrusted foreign trade partners.

One regional free trade agreement that included agriculture was the North American Free Trade Agreement (NAFTA), completed in 1993. This agreement triggered a significant phase-out of agricultural import barriers between the United States and Mexico. For this reason it was strongly opposed by anti-globalization advocacy groups who argued that the agreement would hurt poor corn farmers in Mexico by exposing them to a flood of cheap imports of corn from subsidized growers in the United States. This was later offered as one reason so many Mexican farmers had left the land and moved into urban slums.

Reviewing actual experience since 1993, Mexico did import much more corn from the United States after NAFTA, but this was mostly yellow corn for animal feed to support expanding hog and poultry production, not the white corn for tortillas grown by poor Mexican farmers. Corn production inside Mexico itself actually continued to increase, despite higher imports, in part because commercial corn growers in Mexico were also getting subsidies (37 percent of the income of Mexican corn growers came from government supports in 2002, compared to 26 percent in the United States). A review of academic studies done by the World Bank in 2004 concluded that the decline of Mexican white corn prices was a long-term trend that preceded NAFTA. This study found that the US-Mexico producer price differential for maize did not change significantly after NAFTA came into effect in 1994.

One more recent USDA analysis of 14 US free trade Agreements with a total of 20 countries, revealed that from 1989 through 2020 overall, US agricultural exports to these partner countries increased sixfold, to reach $67.5 billion, while the partner countries saw their agricultural exports to the United States expand as well, more than sixfold, to reach $101.9 billion. During the initial phase-in period, farmers in the partner countries had to make adjustments to greater competition from imports, but they soon found new opportunities to export, typically by turning to higher-value specialty crops.

Lowering import restrictions for basic food staples can nonetheless be a risky policy for some developing countries. Haiti was self-sufficient in rice in the 1970s and 1980s, but in the 1990s it reduced its import tariffs from 50 percent to just 3 percent, allowing less expensive rice from the United States to flood in. Eventually, Haiti was importing 80 percent of its rice and, partly because of lower prices, domestic production stagnated. Then came the international price spike of 2008, which briefly brought a tripling of the import price, followed by riots in the streets of Port-au-Prince. In 2010, former US president Bill Clinton, who was from the rice-growing state of Arkansas, apologized for having supported a set of subsidy and trade policies that helped big farmers in the United States while undercutting small rice producers in Haiti, calling this a "devil's bargain."

Opposition to a reliance on food imports has also been mobilized recently under the banner of "food sovereignty," a social movement that grew up in the 1990s around opposition to agricultural trade liberalization. The lead organization promoting food sovereignty is La Via Campesina (LVC), translated as "the peasant's way." This is a global network of 183 separate local peasant organizations claiming to have at least 200 million members, a somewhat suspect claim since La Via Campesina was not originally a movement led by peasants. It was initially created by anti-globalization activists in Europe, and most of its funding has come from European donors and foundations.

LVC first gained international prominence when it presented a Food Sovereignty manifesto to a forum of more than a thousand NGOs in Rome in 1996. It gained further notoriety in November 1999, when anti-globalization protesters successfully disrupted a WTO ministerial meeting in Seattle, where clashes with riot police left thousands injured and 600 under arrest. In the middle of the street action in Seattle were Central American activists from La Via Campesina, wearing colorful green ball caps and bandanas and demanding food sovereignty. LVC has always had a gift for street theater; at the 1996 Rome meeting, the organization brought truckloads of earth into the city to create a farm field, where supporters engaged in a symbolic planting of seeds.

LVC's food sovereignty vision has evolved over the years toward something increasingly abstract and utopian. In 2007, a Declaration of Nyeleni proclaimed that food sovereignty now meant "new social relations free of oppression and inequality between men and women, peoples, racial groups, social and economic classes and generations." At the core of the food sovereignty vision is resistance not just to international food trade but also to transnational corporate investments and capitalism itself, which LVC depicts as the central threat to peasants. This view skips over the fact that the world's poorest peasants today are found in African countries, like Ethiopia, that attract very little private foreign investment. Outside colonizers of course did terrible damage to poor farmers in regions such as Africa and Latin America, but these colonizers did not arrive as capitalists offering trade and investments. Instead they came as military invaders to steal land, introduce slavery, force conversions to Christianity, and plunder gold and silver.

Do countries that export agricultural products have more political leverage than those that import?

Food exports—especially grain exports—became a more important part of the world's food system after the 1970s. Exports nearly doubled as a share of world grain consumption during that decade alone. This change inspired a view that exporters of grain were gaining increased political leverage over importers. By threatening to reduce or cut off exports, they might be able to exercise international "food power." Arab oil-exporting nations had imposed an embargo on petroleum sales to supporters of the state of Israel to gain leverage, so international strategists speculated that the United States, the world's largest exporter of grains at the time, might be able to secure a parallel strategic advantage by threatening to embargo grain sales.

This presumption was tested in January 1980, when President Jimmy Carter imposed a partial embargo on US grain exports to the Soviet Union to punish them for their recent invasion of Afghanistan. Carter assumed he was in a strong position because at that time the Soviets were expected to import nearly twice as much grain from the United States as they had during the previous 12-month period. If they were prevented from doing so, their use of grains for animal feed—and hence their domestic meat production—might have to be reduced sharply.

In the end this US effort to exercise food power proved to be a failure, because other grain-exporting nations stepped in to provide Moscow with its import needs. Argentina was the first to defy the United States, followed by Australia, and eventually Canada as well. When the Soviet Union offered price premiums to these non-American suppliers, they could not resist. In the end, the Soviet Union imported more grain in 1980, during the embargo, than it had imported in 1979, the year before the embargo. Surprisingly, total US grain exports increased as well during the embargo, when US grain went to the foreign markets abandoned by Argentina, Australia, and Canada. Everyone had changed partners, but all were still dancing. This experience taught an important lesson about the flexibility of international grain markets. When there are multiple suppliers, no one supplier (like the United States) can exercise leverage over importers.

The difficulty of exercising "food power" in international markets was illustrated once again in 2018, when President Donald Trump started a trade war with China by imposing restrictions on imports of Chinese goods, alleging unfair trade practices by Beijing. China retaliated by restricting purchases of US agricultural products, including soybeans and pork. China shifted its purchases to Brazil. The fact that American farmers were the world's leading exporters of these products had not made America powerful; instead it made America vulnerable.

The lesson was learned yet again when Russia invaded Ukraine in 2022, and then began exercising "fuel power" over Europe through sharp cutbacks in its exports of natural gas. Fears arose that Russia would also try to exercise international food power, since Russia and Ukraine respectively accounted for roughly 20 percent and 10 percent of global wheat exports, and together they played a critical role in supplying wheat to markets in the Middle East and North Africa. If Russian naval forces blocked Ukraine's wheat exports through the Black Sea, countries like Egypt might suffer.

Russia and Ukraine did provide a significant share of wheat exports, but together they accounted for only 13 percent of global wheat production, so Egypt was able to meet its needs elsewhere. In June, even before an agreement was reached to unblock food shipments through the Black Sea, Egypt purchased 815,000 metric tons of wheat from France, Bulgaria, Romania, and also from Russia itself (Russia's strategic objective at the time was to coerce Europe, not Egypt).

9

AGRICULTURE AND
THE ENVIRONMENT

Does agriculture always damage the environment?

From the perspective of deep ecology, all forms of agriculture damage the natural environment. When our early ancestors went from hunting and gathering to planting crops and grazing animals, they cut forests and redirected waterways. Wild plants and animals were domesticated, then progressively modified through selective breeding. If preserving nature is the central goal, these actions must be considered damage.

Using a more utilitarian and socially centered perspective, changes to nature caused by farming would be viewed as damage only if they brought long-term costs to human society that exceeded the short-term food production gain. Even under this more forgiving definition, many kinds of farming today clearly do damage the environment.

It is useful to classify the environmental damage done by farming according to where it takes place: on the farm, versus off the farm. Farmers themselves will suffer most from any damage on the farm, while mostly non-farmers pay the price if the damage is off the farm, downstream. In an important way, politics sets the balance between these two kinds of damage. Farmers in poor countries, who lack political power, often find themselves trapped into practices that damage their own farm resource base, and hence their own livelihood. Farmers in rich countries who have considerable political power find it easier to protect their own resource base. They also find it easier to get away with actions that pollute air and water downstream from farms, to the disadvantage of non-farmers.

In the poorest developing countries, most of the environmental damage done by agriculture takes place on the farm itself. Prime examples include the exhaustion of soil nutrients due to shortened fallow times, erosion of soils on sloping lands, the waterlogging of soils due to mismanaged irrigation, and the "desertification" of rangeland caused by excessive animal grazing. By harming the agricultural resource base itself, this sort of damage lowers productivity and helps keep farmers poor. Research presented at an Africa Fertilizer Summit in 2006 revealed that the shortening of fallow times in Africa had removed nitrogen from the soil at an average annual rate of 22–26 kilograms per hectare, far too much to be offset by the prevailing rate of fertilizer application, which then averaged only 9 kilograms per hectare. The result of this "soil mining" was a deficit in soil nutrients that caused annual crop losses estimated at between $1 billion and $3 billion. Nor was this the end of the problem. As cultivated soils become exhausted, farmers will extend cropping onto new lands, cutting more trees and destroying more wildlife habitat. According to the World Resources Institute, land clearing for the expansion of unsustainable low-yield farming has caused roughly 70 percent of all deforestation in Africa.

In wealthy industrial societies, by contrast, environmental damage from farming usually results from too much input use rather than too little, and those who suffer most are usually not farmers. For example, excessive nitrogen fertilizer use leads to nitrate runoff and eutrophication of streams and ponds. In Europe, excess nitrates in water are a downstream health hazard ("blue baby syndrome"). In the United States, excessive nitrogen fertilizer use on farms in the Mississippi River watershed contributes to an environmental calamity both within that watershed and also in the Gulf of Mexico, where by

2017 an 8,776 square mile "dead zone" no longer able to support aquatic life had formed at the mouth of the Mississippi River. In the Florida Everglades, nitrogen and phosphorus runoff from sugarcane production has produced cattail growth so thick as to replace the native sawgrass, ruining the habitat of wading birds like storks, and sucking oxygen from the water when the cattails die and decompose, which kills the fish.

Exploitation of river water for crop irrigation can also harm migratory fish species, such as salmon, which are unable to move upstream through the narrow passages and turbines of dams. Concentrated animal feeding operations (CAFOs), designed to cut livestock industry costs by fattening thousands of animals for slaughter within large crowded facilities, can pollute both the air and water with toxic effluents, creating health risks for non-farming human populations living nearby. The poultry industry in just a single county in Delaware produces 200 million birds a year, and mishandled chicken waste has been a major source of eutrophication in the Chesapeake Bay.

What kind of farming is environmentally sustainable?

Environmental activists and agricultural scientists answer this question in dramatically different ways. Environmentalists usually prefer small-scale diversified farming systems that rely on fewer inputs purchased off the farm, and on systems that imitate nature rather than trying to engineer or dominate nature. Agricultural scientists, in contrast, tend to assume that there will be less harm done to nature overall by moving toward specialized high-yield farming systems employing the latest technology, since increasing crop yields on lands already being farmed will allow more of the remaining land to be saved for nature. While environmentalists invoke the damage done by modern farming, agricultural scientists invoke the greater damage that would be done if today's volume of production had to come from low-yield farming systems. Compared to 1948, farms in the United States today are producing three times as much output. If we had tried to triple production using the farming methods of 1948, the environmental damage today would be far greater.

The environmentalist side of this argument took some of its early inspiration from Rachel Carson's 1962 book, *Silent Spring*, which exposed the damage done by chemical pesticides both to human health and to wild animal species (including songbirds, hence the title). Carson's book led to a legal ban on the agricultural use of DDT in the United States and also to the formation of a broad and powerful environmental movement, which in 1970 secured passage of the National Environmental Protection Act, creating America's Environmental Protection Agency (EPA).

Carson's thinking inspired a continuing quest among environmentalists to find alternatives to high-yield "industrial" farming. One early pioneer in this search was Wes Jackson, who founded a Land Institute in Kansas in 1976, to promote farming based on polycultures of perennial crops rather than monocultures of annual crops. This approach did not prove to be a commercial success, but it was Jackson, in 1980, who began employing the term "sustainable agriculture" to describe his goal. Responding to political interest in alternative farming systems, the US Department of Agriculture (USDA) in 1985 finally initiated a program to promote what it called low-impact sustainable agriculture, or LISA. Conventional commercial farmers panned it as "low income sustainable agriculture," but the idea gained traction with non-farming urban populations and with a younger cohort of countercultural farmers who had links to a back-to-the-land movement from the 1960s.

High-yield farming did cause environmental damage in America during the second half of the twentieth century, but the earlier style of low-yield farming had also been damaging. It was an extension of low-yield wheat farming into the southern plains of Kansas, Oklahoma, and the Texas panhandle in the 1920s, before synthetic chemical fertilizers or pesticides were in wide use, that produced America's single greatest environmental disaster at that time, a drought-induced loss of topsoil that ruined farmlands across an area as big as the state of Pennsylvania, turning it into a "dust bowl." Roughly 400,000 farmers fled the dust bowl, many of them moving to California to work as migrants picking tomatoes and peas. This was a flow of environmental refugees unmatched for seven decades, until Hurricane Katrina subsequently flooded out the population of New Orleans in 2005.

Following Carson's book, while environmentalists were concluding that chemical use to increase crop yields was inherently dangerous, commercial farmers and agricultural scientists sought instead to develop new chemicals that were less harmful, and they looked for ways to apply them with greater precision to reduce runoff. Environmental advocates were not impressed with this "technical fix" approach; they wanted a more complete move away from highly specialized, highly capitalized "industrial" farming. Their views were later supported by a 2008 International Assessment of Agricultural Science and Technology for Development (IAASTD), which warned that using still more modern science to "increase yields and productivity" could do even more environmental damage.

Growing numbers of popular writers have embraced this view. In an apocalyptic 2008 book titled *The End of Food*, journalist Paul Roberts argued that the world's large-scale, hyper-efficient industrialized food production systems were heading toward an inevitable collapse because of the damage they had been doing to soils, water systems, and other "natural infrastructure." In 2013, *New York Times* food columnist Mark Bittman described America's "hyper-industrial" agricultural system as having poisoned land and water, wasted energy, and made a major contribution to climate change. "We must figure out a way to un-invent this food system," said Bittman. Despite such popular sentiments, a preponderance of agricultural scientists and economists do not reject today's large-scale, specialized, and highly capitalized farming systems as unsustainable. In fact, they view these systems as the best means available to contain environmental damage from farming, given today's much larger production requirements.

What is "precision agriculture"?

Commercial farming today has moved well beyond the indiscriminate chemical use that Rachel Carson properly criticized in 1962. Many of the early insecticides then in use have now been banned and replaced by chemicals that are less persistent in the environment and effective when applied in lower volume. Commercial farmers are always looking for ways to cut back on unnecessary chemical and fuel use so as to reduce input costs, and by the end of the 20th century they had found a number of technical means to do so. These new methods came to be labeled "precision agriculture" (PA).

Beginning in the 1970s and 1980s, during an interlude of extremely high energy prices, farmers in the United States first learned to save diesel fuel by planting seeds in unplowed fields—a "no-till" approach to farming that also reduced erosion, conserved soil moisture, and sequestered carbon. They also switched from flood irrigation to less wasteful center-pivot sprays, and to laser-leveled fields with zero runoff, and also to more precise drip irrigation systems. Then, in the 1990s, they began using Global Positioning Systems (GPS) to auto-steer tractors in perfectly straight lines with zero overlap (saving more diesel fuel), plus digital soil-mapping and onboard computer systems to match chemical applications of fertilizer or lime more precisely to location-specific needs. GPS satellites, when supported by on-farm base stations that send correction signals to the machinery in the field, can locate that machinery in real time with sub-inch accuracy. With variable-rate application capabilities, these machines can deliver precisely the amount of water or fertilizer required at that location in the field. Infrared sensors can be used to detect the greenness of a crop, telling a farmer exactly how much more (or less) fertilizer might be needed. To minimize nitrogen runoff, fertilizer can also be dripped into the soil in much smaller total quantities and in perfect rows exactly where the seeds will be planted. Modern commercial farms also make use of imaging from unmanned aerial vehicles (UAV), artificial intelligence (AI), robotics, machine learning, and big data. Since the 1990s, farmers in the United States also began planting genetically engineered soybean, corn, and cotton seeds that made it possible to control weeds without mechanical tillage and to control insects without as many chemical sprays.

Farmers took up these more precise methods to save money on chemicals, water, and diesel fuel, but the side result was a clear benefit to the environment. American agricultural output has increased by 45 percent since the early 1980s, but chemical fertilizer use has remained flat in absolute terms, and the total pounds of pesticide applied to American crops actually declined by 18 percent in absolute terms between 1980 and 2008. Insecticide use, specifically, has now fallen more than 80 percent from its 1972 peak. Thanks to higher yields, land use has been reduced as well. American farms are planting 20 percent less land to corn today than they were in 1940, even though total corn production has increased fivefold. Modern corn production saves more than just land; for every bushel of corn produced since 1980, the use of irrigation water has fallen 46 percent, energy use 41 percent, and greenhouse gas emissions 31 percent.

One important innovation in modern crop farming has been "conservation tillage," which includes not plowing the soil at all ("no till"), or plowing only narrow strips in a field ("strip till"), or leaving crop residues on at least one-third of the soil ("mulch till"). Originally adopted to save on diesel fuel, these methods also reduce soil erosion, help retain soil moisture, and sequester carbon in the ground. In 2022, the USDA reported that American farmers were employing some form of conservation tillage on 68 percent of wheat acres, 74 percent of soybean acres, and 76 percent of corn acres. As of 2022, American farmers were planting cover crops on 40 percent of their land to protect their soil during the winter months.

Modern livestock farming has also become less damaging to the environment. Today's livestock systems urgently need tighter regulation on animal welfare grounds, but when it comes to environmental protection they actually perform better than traditional methods for every pound of food produced. Consider dairy farms. Modern cow confinement systems can be objectionable on animal welfare grounds compared to traditional pasturing, but they require 94 percent less human labor for every gallon of milk production, 90 percent less land, two-thirds less feed and water, and—most surprising of all—79 percent fewer animals.

Likewise for pork production, since average feed requirements for every added pound of weight gain in pigs has fallen almost by half since the 1990s. For chickens since 1950, average feed requirements per pound of live-weight broilers declined more than one-third. Compared to the 1970s, every pound of beef production now requires 12 percent less water, 19 percent less feed, 30 percent fewer animals, and 33 percent less land, and it generates 18 percent less manure.

Environmental damage continues to be done by America's farms, but this damage has been driven not by how we farm but instead by how much more we must produce today to satisfy consumer demands, particularly for animal products. Total meat consumption in the United States today is five times as high as it was in 1940, creating an environmental burden that even our most efficient and precise farming systems cannot fully contain. America's biggest environmental policy challenge in farming today may be to change the way we eat, not the way we farm.

The United States has not been alone in using new technology to move commercial farming toward a reduced use of inputs per bushel of production. In 2008 the Organisation for Economic Co-operation and Development (OECD) in Paris published an important review of the "environmental

performance of agriculture" in the 30 most advanced industrial countries of the world (those with the most specialized
and most highly capitalized farming systems). The new data
showed that between 1990 and 2004, total food production in
these countries increased in volume by 5 percent from an already high level, yet adverse environmental impacts had diminished in nearly every category. The area of land taken up
by agriculture declined 4 percent. Soil erosion from both wind
and water was reduced. Water use on irrigated lands declined
by 9 percent. Energy use on the farm increased at only one-sixth
the rate of energy use in the rest of the economy. Gross greenhouse gas emissions from farming fell by 3 percent. Herbicide
and insecticide spraying declined by 5 percent. Excessive nitrogen fertilizer use declined by 17 percent. Biodiversity also
improved, as increased numbers of crop varieties and livestock breeds came into use.

The precision farming vision is embraced by so-called
eco-modernists who believe scientific innovation is the best
way to decouple wealth creation from environmental harm,
but traditional environmentalists, including Green parties
in Europe, prefer a return to premodern methods, including
organic farming, which uses no synthetic fertilizer at all. As
mentioned in Chapter 8, European Greens in 2019 pushed the
EU to embrace a European Green Deal, including a "Farm to
Fork" strategy for agriculture designed to triple organic crop
acreage by 2030, while using Europe's influence through trade
and assistance agreements to nudge other countries in the
same direction. In 2021 the US Secretary of Agriculture, Tom
Vilsack, pushed back against the EU by announcing the formation of an Agriculture Innovation Mission for Climate (AIM
for Climate) initiative, and a Sustainable Productivity Growth
Coalition (SPG) of governments, agencies, foundations, research organizations, and private companies committed to a
more innovation-based, science-forward path.

True believers in the promise of precision farming expect
there will be no end to the environmental gains that can be

achieved. Their long-term vision includes small solar-powered robots working farm fields using multi-camera arrays and powerful algorithms to recognize and eliminate weeds and bugs 24 hours a day, burning no fossil fuels and using almost no polluting chemicals. Even if this fantasy becomes possible, traditional environmental advocates will probably refuse to see it as progress. They generally do not endorse modern precision farming, since it favors highly capitalized industrial-scale operations that they reject on principle. The small, diversified farms they prefer cannot make use of the costly machinery that is a key component to most modern precision farming. In addition, environmental advocates instinctively reject the notion that biological systems based on plants and animals can be sustainably managed through industrial methods, using digital science. They believe, with Carson, that nature will always find a way to strike back against this kind of human arrogance.

Do fragile lands, population growth, and poverty make farming unsustainable?

These are popular explanations for environmental damage from farming, but the damage usually comes instead from faulty human institutions.

For example, supposedly "fragile" lands in tropical countries do not have to degrade or erode, even sloping or irregular lands with thin and badly weathered soils subject to damaging extremes of heat, flood, and drought. When poorly managed, if soil nutrients are not replaced, such lands will soon become a barren landscape on which only weeds will grow. But under proper management, these less productive tropical lands can be improved dramatically and farmed sustainably. When farmed with adequate fallow time, or treated with lime to the correct acidity, or terraced and mulched to capture and keep more moisture on leveled soil, or planted to several different crops at the same time (intercropped) to reduce vulnerability to pests, the productive potential of such less-favored lands can be sustainably increased.

Some argue that poverty itself is a cause of environmental damage in farming, because poor farmers who live from hand to mouth cannot afford to wait for resource-protecting investments to pay off. Yet many poor farming communities will invest a great deal to protect their resources, so long as the political and institutional circumstances are right. They are more than willing to build and maintain terraces, plant trees, and protect rangelands from overgrazing when effective "common property resource" (CPR) systems are allowed to operate at the local or village level. These informal systems protect local forests, streams, ponds, and grazing lands by allocating equitable rights of use to insiders while denying access to outsiders. Such systems are good at blocking the "tragedy of the commons," a pattern of environmental destruction that arises in systems of open access (Garrett Hardin, the influential ecologist who named this danger in 1968, should have called it the "tragedy of open access"). Within well-managed commons systems, even poor communities can avoid environmental tragedies.

Effective CPR systems are vulnerable to breakdown, however, if powerful outside institutions, such as colonial administrators, international companies, forestry department bureaucrats, megaproject engineers, government land-titling agencies, or centralized irrigation authorities move in to take control away from local community leaders. Local farmers who sense they are about to lose control of their resource base will at that point stop making investments in resource protection. They will begin using up the resource as fast as they can— cutting the trees, plowing up terraces, overgrazing the range, overfishing the ponds—before the outsiders take it away completely. Poor farmers who have control as well as access can be conserving farmers, but if control is taken away they will use their access to exploit rather than conserve.

Well-functioning common property systems in poor countries can also break down due to rapid population growth. If population density increases beyond a certain point, the value gained per person from protecting the resource will decline for insiders (demotivating protection efforts), and this will happen just at the time when many more outsiders are attempting to gain access. At this point, effective resource protection can require switching to a stronger individual private property system, one that restores payoffs for individual resource-protecting actions and hands the problem of excluding outsiders over to the police. If this transition to individual land ownership is successfully made, a further increase in population density need not threaten the resource base at all. In fact, greater population density makes affordable greater labor investments in protecting the land (mulching, terracing, etc.) while also increasing the human payoff from productivity-enhancing rural public goods investments in roads, power, and irrigation.

One example from Africa is the experience of the Machakos District in Kenya, where farmers in this densely settled semi-arid area avoided serious damage to their marginal soil endowments even as population increased. This occurred thanks to clearly titled land ownership that motivated heavier labor investments in terracing systems, use of more fertilizer, and a shift to higher-value crops for sale in nearby urban markets.

Do cash crops and export crops cause environmental harm?

Shifting from food crop production to a more specialized cash crop production for export has frequently been cited as a cause of both economic dependency and environmental harm. There are some cases that support this generalization, for example in Central America in the 1960s and 1970s, when landlords introduced chemical-intensive cotton production and evicted traditional peasants growing maize and beans. Yet the cash crop versus food crop dichotomy is usually misleading, because a number of food crops in the developing world are at the same time cash crops (for example, rice in Asia), and many cash export crops (such as cocoa in West Africa) are grown by small farmers in the same fields with food crops in an environmentally friendly intercropping system.

Cash crops for export are not inherently less rewarding for small farmers to grow, nor are they inherently more damaging to the environment. Exported cash crops are often tree crops or perennials that provide better land cover and more stable root structures compared to annual food crops. In Africa, some kinds of perennial export crops—such as tea or coffee, planted along the contour of sloping lands, or oil palm planted in low-lying areas—can protect the soil much better than food crops such as maize, requiring annual tillage. A partial switch to higher-value cash crops also helps farm families with limited land and labor earn the income they need to purchase food between harvests, and also to pay for their children's school expenses. When farmers switch part of their land to cash crop production, they also can use some of the income to purchase improved seeds and fertilizer, simultaneously boosting food crop production on the rest of their land.

Do farm subsidies promote environmental damage in agriculture?

Often they do. Subsidy policies that give farmers artificially high prices per bushel for their products will induce an excessive use of fertilizers, pesticides, and irrigation water, because the marginal cost of more input use will be more than offset by a higher marginal return for every added bushel. In Japan, where farmers enjoy high border protections, especially for rice, pesticide use is high at 11 kilograms per hectare of cropland. In the United States with lower protection levels, crop farmers use only 2.5 kilograms per hectare. In Ethiopia, where farmers get almost no protection at all, pesticide use averages only 0.2 kilograms per hectare. In most of Africa, farmers are often taxed rather than subsidized (a symptom of their political weakness), which frequently results in too little chemical use rather than too much. Fertilizer use in much of Africa is insufficient to replace the soil nutrients taken up by crops.

Sometimes governments subsidize chemical use directly, partly as a way to help farmers and partly to help government-owned chemical companies. In Indonesia in the 1980s, when the government subsidized farm purchases of fertilizer by as much as 68 percent, chemical use increased 77 percent over one five-year period. Governments also indirectly subsidize water use. In India, when the government began to subsidize 86 percent of the electric bill for pumping irrigation water in the Punjab, groundwater tables began dropping at an unsustainable rate of about 0.8 meters a year.

In rich countries, farmers are not only powerful enough politically to demand the subsidies that encourage excessive input use, they are also powerful enough to avoid being held accountable for the resulting downstream environmental damage. Because of farm lobby strength, the air and water pollution that emanates from farms in rich countries is regulated far less than pollution from other industries. In the United States, the agricultural sector is significantly exempt from the regulatory structures of both the original Clean Air Act and Clean Water Act, because pollution from farms does not come from a "point source."

Despite the dead zone in the Gulf of Mexico, Congress does not regulate excess nitrogen runoff from farms and does not tax farm fertilizer use. Instead, it has created voluntary programs that pay farmers to take land (temporarily) out of production, or to cultivate their land in ways that reduce runoff. These incentive-based, voluntary conservation programs operated by the USDA have recently cost taxpayers roughly $5.4 billion per year. Instead of using a "polluter pays" principle, the government pays farmers to do a better job of protecting their own land. Even in extreme cases such as chemical pollution in the Florida Everglades from heavily subsidized sugar farming, strong regulations are routinely blocked by the industry. In 1996, when Vice President Al Gore proposed taxing sugar growers to finance an Everglades clean-up project, a direct phone call from a Florida sugar baron to President Bill Clinton resulted in the tax proposal's being set aside.

The power of agricultural interests to resist environmental regulation has also been seen in climate policy. In 2009, when the House of Representatives passed the Waxman-Markey bill to create a cap-and-trade system to limit greenhouse gas emissions, the entire agricultural sector was left "uncapped." Instead of being subject to caps under this bill, farmers would have been entitled to profit by selling "offsets" to industries in sectors that were capped. The offset would be based on a voluntary reduction in emissions, or an increased sequestering of carbon—things a farmer might be doing anyway, or might be doing just temporarily.

Commercial farmers in the United States continue to fight political battles with environmental regulators at the Environmental Protection Agency (EPA). One long-running dispute has been over various federal water protection rules on farms. In 2015, when the Obama administration attempted to expand water management rules to include ditches that "look and act" like water tributaries, as well as to any body of water within 1,500 feet of another water body already covered by the rules, farmers raised loud objections, out of fear that they would now need government permits to dig ditches on their own land. Under pressure from farm groups, 28 states successfully sought injunctions to block the expanded rules, which the Trump administration repealed in 2019 and 2020. The issue continues to be a political football.

One of the few environmental policy instruments strong enough to resist the farm lobby in the United States has been the 1973 Endangered Species Act. For example, in 2008, a lawsuit filed under that act by the Natural Resources Defense

Council forced the Bush administration's Fish and Wildlife Service to divert more than 150 billion gallons of water away from irrigated farming in the San Joaquin Valley, in California, so as to protect the delta smelt, an endangered 3-inch bait fish. Environmentalists know that their best chance, in a battle against farmers, is usually to move the action out of Congress and into the courts.

How will climate change affect food production?

In 2022, the surface temperature of the earth was 1.55 degrees F warmer than the twentieth-century average of 57.0 degrees F. The current period is now the warmest in the history of modern civilization, but the impacts on agriculture are complex and mostly site-specific. In the tropics, higher temperatures in the future will pose a serious threat to farming, since some crops are already being grown near the upper range of their biological heat tolerance, but in some high-latitude temperate zone regions, warmer weather will mean longer growing seasons and perhaps the chance to plant a second annual crop. Average rainfall and rainfall variability will change as well, but in ways far more difficult to predict. A warming earth will be, on average, a wetter earth, due to accelerated ocean evaporation leading to increased cloud formation, and in some places this may be good for farming. Increased carbon dioxide (CO_2) in the atmosphere can also help farming, since plants need to take in CO_2. This is known as the carbon fertilization effect. But increased atmospheric ozone, another greenhouse gas, can slow plant growth.

In North America, longer growing seasons at upper latitudes, more rainfall overall, and greater carbon fertilization may actually provide net benefits to farming. According to one early estimate from the Intergovernmental Panel on Climate Change (IPCC), crop yields in North America were expected to increase by 5–20 percent during the first several decades of the 21st century, due to climate change. At the same time, these gains were expected to be uneven across the region, and weather variations were likely to be more extreme. Since the beginning of the last century, annual precipitation has increased across most of the northern and eastern United States but decreased across much of the southern and western parts of the country. Over the coming century, significant increases in precipitation are projected in winter and spring over the Northern Great Plains, the Upper Midwest, and the Northeast. Experts still disagree on whether the severe 2012 summer drought in the United States was linked more to long-term climate change versus to short-term factors such as a cyclical La Niña effect.

The impacts of climate change on farming in the developing world are almost certain to be more damaging. One 2009 projection done by the International Food Policy Research Institute (IFPRI) was based on a linked computer model that incorporated both a food supply-and-demand component and a biological crop growth component, estimating yield changes driven by temperature changes within 281 different spatial regions around the world. The temperature changes expected within these spatial regions, out to the year 2050, were calculated based on modeled scenarios generated from the IPCC's 2007 4th Assessment Report. The results of this exercise were alarming. Rice production in the developing world in 2050 was expected to be 14 percent lower with climate change compared to without, and due to climate change wheat production in the developing world was expected to be 34 percent lower than it would have been otherwise. In South Asia, specifically, wheat production was projected to be 49 percent lower in a 2050 world with climate change, compared to a world without climate change. When IFPRI then put these projected production impacts into its economic model, it was able to estimate the higher food prices these climate effects would generate and concluded that there would be a 23 percent increase in the numbers of malnourished children expected in 2050 in a world with climate change, compared to a world without.

In response to such threats, food producers will likely prioritize strategies of adaptation, through investments in things like irrigation, which builds local resilience quickly. "Mitigation" strategies to reduce greenhouse gas emissions from food production, or to sequester carbon in the ground, are good for the longer run, but average temperatures will continue increasing over the next several decades even if global emissions are reduced, so adaptation will remain a short-run imperative even if mitigation can eventually be successful. This is especially true for countries in the tropics where farming faces the largest climate threat.

Adapting food systems to climate change will require large investments in infrastructure, such as cold chains in food marketing and irrigation, plus agricultural R&D to develop drought- and heat-tolerant crops. IFPRI calculated in 2009 that if an added $7 billion were properly spent on irrigation, rural roads, and agricultural research, the adverse impacts of climate change on food production might be offset. At the time this seemed a relatively small amount, but raising money in rich countries for climate adaptation investments in poor countries is politically challenging, since nearly all the benefits are captured in those poor countries. Today's rich countries are responsible for most of the emissions that created the problem, and at a climate summit in Copenhagen in 2009 they pledged $100 billion a year in climate finance for poor countries, to be balanced between mitigation and adaptation, but they fell far short in honoring this pledge. An independent analysis by Oxfam a decade later concluded that in 2017–2018 only about $20 billion was provided, and only a quarter of that went for adaptation, and just a small fraction of this adaptation funding went to the agricultural sector. One 2021 report found that, globally, just 0.2 percent of all tracked climate-related financing went to small holder farmers.

So far, thanks to past investments in agricultural science and infrastructure, most high-resource farmers in the more prosperous societies have been able to stay ahead of the climate threat. Crop yields in the OECD region as a whole not only remain high; they keep going up. For these 38 countries, wheat yields today are 22 percent higher than they were in 1990, and corn yields are 51 percent higher. This has come from strong resource investments in better seeds and irrigation where necessary. Even in the drought-threatened countries of East Africa, FAO data show that per capita agricultural production managed to increase 15 percent between 2000 and 2010. But subsequently it increased only by another 1 percent between 2010 and 2020, and too much of this production increase was achieved through a damaging and unsustainable expansion of low-yield farming onto dry lands or into forest land. This increases future vulnerability to drought, destroys wildlife habitat, and threatens biodiversity.

Can we reduce agriculture's contribution to climate change?

Agriculture is not only affected by climate change; farming and ranching activities are themselves a significant source of greenhouse gas emissions. In the United States, the agricultural sector accounted for 11.2 percent of total US greenhouse gas emissions in 2020. World-wide, agriculture emits roughly 18 percent of the global total. The exact mix of greenhouse gas emissions differs between rich and poor. In the United States, half of all direct agricultural emissions consist of nitrous oxide, about 70 percent of that from fertilizer. Much of the rest is methane from ruminant animals. Electricity use and direct carbon dioxide emissions account for only a bit more than 10 percent of the agricultural total. In developing countries, a much larger share of greenhouse gas emissions comes from land use changes, particularly from clearing trees and cutting bush to create more crop and pasture land, releasing carbon dioxide when the trees are burned and the soil plowed. Such emissions have slowed in Asia and South America thanks to a slowing of deforestation, but between 2000 and 2018, emissions in Africa continued to rise as cropland area continued to increase. During the 2000–2018 period, Africa's agricultural emissions increased to constitute 24 percent of world agricultural total, up from 18 percent in 2000.

The best way to slow land conversions to farming in regions like Africa is to increase crop yields on land already being farmed, through bigger investments in irrigation, fertilizer, and improved seeds. In rich countries the parallel strategy would be to speed the progress being made toward precision farming methods, particularly to reduce excessive fertilizer use. In the livestock and dairy sectors, as noted above, considerable progress has already been made in reducing greenhouse gas emissions for every pound of production. By one 2019 calculation made by Frank Mitloehner, a professor of animal science and an air quality specialist at the University of California, Davis, the climate burden of a single glass of milk in the United States today is actually two-thirds smaller than it was 70 years ago.

One embarrassing truth about America's greenhouse gas emissions from agriculture is not so much the damage caused by how we farm, but the damage caused by how much we eat, especially animal products. Meat consumption in the United States today is five times as high as it was in 1940. Red meat consumption, from ruminant animals like cattle that burp out methane from their second stomach, has been coming down in America on a per capita basis, but it remains much too high both for personal health and for climate health. One 2019 study by the EAT-Lancet Commission found that Americans would have to eat 84 percent less red meat to stay within both health-protection and climate-protection boundaries.

Some advocates have recently come to believe that crop farming and animal production could actually help mitigate climate, if a transition could be made to "regenerative" methods. They claim that properly managed soils, in farm fields and pastures, can store carbon underground after removing it from the atmosphere through the natural process of photosynthesis. For crops, the favored regenerative methods are no-till farming and planting cover crops in the winter months; for animals the recommended method is rotational grazing, which moves animals in groups from place to place to give the pasture grass time to enjoy vigorous growth. One of the most prominent advocates for regenerative agriculture in the United States has become Al Gore, the former vice president, who employs these methods on his own farm in Carthage, Tennessee, where he convenes "Carbon Underground" meetings to promote the idea.

No-till cropping, cover crops, and rotational grazing can all make sense for improving soil and pasture health, but scientists do not yet agree on how much carbon dioxide these methods can remove permanently from the atmosphere. The sequestration gains from cropping might only be temporary if a field is plowed again, and for cattle grazing the sequestration gains would have to be very large to offset the added methane emissions that come from grazed animals, since it takes them a longer time to reach a market weight compared to cattle in feedlots. By most standard calculations, feedlot beef has a climate burden 18.5–67.5 percent lower than fully grass-fed beef.

The carbon sequestration claims made by the regenerative agriculture movement have so far been hard to either prove or disprove, because the measurement problem is so difficult. Soil conditions can differ every 10 feet or so, as well as at different depths. The sampling and testing required simply to establish a confident carbon content baseline is too expensive for use at scale.

These measurement problems contributed, in 2021, to an early decision by the Biden administration not to create a "carbon bank" inside USDA to broker the selling of "carbon credits" from regenerative farmers to private companies that needed help in meeting their emissions reduction pledges. Biden had floated this idea during his 2020 campaign, but one senior editor at the *MIT Technology Review* raised a warning, saying it could become a phony solution, with companies claiming unverified credits from farmers for carbon sequestration that might only be temporary, while avoiding cutting emissions from their own operations.

The Biden administration decided instead in 2022 to launch a $3 billion grant program, to fund peer-reviewed pilot studies conducted by farm groups, universities, and local governments to show which farming practices could deliver measurable "climate smart" results. As the results come in, specific practices can be classified as "climate smart" and farms adopting these practices can sell their products with a "climate smart" label. Climate-conscious shoppers in the market will then reward these farmers by paying a premium price.

Will expanded irrigation harm the environment?

For crop and livestock farmers everywhere, fresh water is an essential resource. Producing 1 kilogram of wheat requires the use of about 1,000 liters of water, and paddy rice requires twice this amount. Larger investments in irrigation would seem to be one way to adapt to the more severe droughts expected to accompany climate change. In the developing world today, while irrigated land makes up only one-fifth of total arable area, it supports two-fifths of all crop production including close to three-fifths of all cereals. Yet poorly managed irrigation systems can also damage the environment. Is there room for them to expand in a sustainable fashion the future?

In the past 60 years, irrigated area has more than doubled and now accounts for 22 percent of global cropland. A 2022 study published in *Environmental Research* showed that much of this expansion took place during the early years of the Green Revolution, when abundant and dependable water supplies were needed to take full advantage of the new seeds. This expansion of irrigated area has continued; between 2000 and 2019, irrigated area increased by an additional 18 percent. Still more expansion, particularly in Africa, would be good for reducing climate vulnerability and increasing farm productivity, but it may not be easy to achieve.

Continuing to expand the use of irrigation water for agriculture will be difficult for several reasons. First, the most promising sites for irrigation have already been developed. Second is growing competition for freshwater use by urban dwellers and industries. Third will be the unfortunate degradation of some past irrigation sites. Poor drainage of irrigated lands has left some waterlogged or saline. Basins behind dams have silted up, reducing capacity. In many large rivers, excessive withdrawals have left as little as 5 percent of the former water volume in-stream, and some rivers no longer reach the sea year-round.

Building river dams, either for power or irrigation, also encounters opposition from environmental groups. Because so many non-governmental organizations (NGOs) are now opposed to dams, the World Bank has virtually stopped financing such projects in the developing world. NGOs tend to favor small-scale irrigation alternatives such as rainwater harvesting, bucket irrigation, treadle and pedal pumps, and small earthen dams, yet these options are hard to scale up and they carry excessive labor costs in much of rural Africa. Citizens in today's rich countries gained prosperity in part by building dams to develop 70 percent or more of their own hydroelectric potential, so they should think twice before telling Africa—where only 3 percent of potential has so far been developed—that dams are a bad idea.

Nearly 40 percent of irrigated area now depends primarily on groundwater, yet aquifer depletion is a growing threat in regions like South Asia because rates of pumping have proved nearly impossible to regulate. In one 2012 estimate published in *Nature*, roughly 1.7 billion people were living in areas where groundwater resources or groundwater-dependent ecosystems were under threat.

In Africa, however, groundwater resources have been underexploited. A 2022 study conducted by the British Geological Survey concluded that most African countries had sufficient groundwater, along with a sufficient annual recharge rate from rainfall, to allow sustainable pumping both for personal consumption and for the irrigation of high-value agricultural crops. Currently, only 4 percent of cropland in Sub-Saharan Africa is irrigated, compared to 37 percent in Asia.

Governments have historically preferred to invest in surface water irrigation schemes rather than groundwater pumping, because pumped groundwater tends to remain in private hands beyond governmental control. With so many African farmers at increasing risk of drought due to climate change, it seems a mistake to allow their rechargeable groundwater resources to go untapped.

What can be done to improve water management in farming?

The first and most important step is to reduce water waste. The technical means available include shifting from flood irrigation to more precise spray or drip systems, leveling fields with lasers to eliminate runoff, and lining irrigation canals to reduce seepage. The policy steps needed include ending subsidies for cheap electricity that encourage excessive pumping (e.g., in India), establishing water users' associations to regulate access, and creating water markets based on tradeable water rights.

Private water markets have saved farming in some dry parts of Australia. One example is the Murray-Darling Basin, where the Australian government in the 1990s shifted from building dams and subsidizing water to a policy that separated water rights from land rights. This allowed farmers with less need for water to sell their rights to farmers who needed more. Total water availability was falling in this basin, yet the income of farmers remained high, thanks to the operation of this water market. As water availability went down, the price of water went up, which encouraged growers of low-value water-demanding crops such as rice to sell some of their water rights to growers of higher-value crops such as vegetables or grapes. The system allows willing buyers and willing sellers to make deals that allocate scarce water to its highest value use. Water trading systems for farmers also operate at the state level in the western part of the United States, in Arizona, New Mexico, Colorado, and California.

In California, new precision farming techniques have been developed to reduce water waste in almond production. This one state produces 82 percent of all the almonds in the world, and every year each acre of almond trees uses 3–4 acre-feet of water (one acre of water a foot deep), which is not sustainable in California's water-stressed Central Valley. Almond growers have long used drip irrigation to reduce water waste, but these systems are now being made "smart" with sensors in the soil that can deliver continuous moisture readings, telling the water to drip at a variable rate location by location, only as much as needed. On one operation the farm manager has divided his almond groves into smaller blocks, each separately irrigated through smart drip lines linked electronically to soil moisture probes that send data back to the "brain" of the system by radio signal. The data indicate moisture levels both by location and soil depth, and are continuously relayed to a mobile app used by the farm manager. Instead of putting on water 24 hours a day, the drip lines can operate block-by-block only as needed.

Variable rate irrigation systems of this kind can now be integrated into conventional systems simply by adding the appropriate controllers and software. A setup can be costly because it is custom-tailored to each crop on each farm, but as equipment manufacturers develop better standards to facilitate ease of set up, ease of use, and interchangeability, the uptake of such systems will increase, not just for almonds and not just in California.

10

LIVESTOCK, MEAT, AND FISH

How are farm animals different from crops?

In some respects, they are not so different. Human beings have eaten animals—including fish—from the beginning, and we have bred domesticated animals to serve our food purposes in much the way that we have bred crop plants. Moreover, market forces are pushing modern livestock production systems and modern crop production systems in roughly the same capital-intensive and information-intensive direction, leading to increased specialization, mechanization, and automation, all to reduce land and labor requirements. Consumer prices for animal products have fallen over the long term, parallel to the long-term decline in crop prices.

In at least four respects, however, farm animals are significantly different from crop plants. First, and most obviously, animals tend to move around, making their management more complicated. Second, they must be managed according to a much higher ethical standard, because unlike plants they have complex social and emotional lives that should command our respect. After all, we ourselves are animals. Third, farm animals must themselves be given food, often several times a day and in large amounts, making the food products we get from animals more costly both to consumers and the environment. Fourth, farm animals produce manure, which is a valuable product for restoring soil nutrients if managed properly, but if mismanaged it becomes a human health hazard and a damaging source of water and air pollution.

Is meat consumption increasing, or not?

Global meat consumption has tripled over the last 50 years, and it continues to rise annually at a rapid 3.5 percent rate, meaning it could double once more in the next two decades. To sustain this higher consumption, herders and livestock producers around the world are now managing three times as many domesticated food animals as the earth has people. Globally, a surprising 73 percent of all these food animals are chickens. Total meat consumption has also continued to increase in the United States, even on a per capita basis. It appeared to be peaking at 272 pounds annually in 2006, but after a brief dip it reached a new peak at 278 pounds in 2019. One encouraging change in the American diet has been a shift toward poultry consumption and away from ruminant animal products such as beef and dairy products, which cause methane emissions. On a per capita basis, beef consumption in the United States peaked in 1976, and by 2019 it had fallen by 21 percent.

The driving factors behind the global increase in raising animals for food have been human population growth and personal income growth. As societies become more wealthy, people almost invariably use a part of the higher income to purchase more meat, milk, and eggs. China illustrates this tendency. In the 1960s when China was still a poor country, the average person consumed less than 5 kilograms of meat annually. But when incomes grew following China's market-driven reforms in the late 1970s, consumption rose to 20 kilograms per capita by the late 1980s. It has now grown to 63 kilograms, especially pork. China now consumes half of all the world's pork. In most rich countries, meat consumption per person is no longer increasing, but in the transitional countries of Asia and Latin America it still has considerable room to grow, and even more in the poor countries of Africa. According to one projection by the International Food Policy Research Institute, between 2010 and 2050 per capita meat consumption in Latin America is likely to rise by 33 percent, in East Asia and the Pacific by 86 percent, and in Sub-Saharan Africa by 118 percent (but from a much lower level). Rich countries are the big meat consumers today, but in the decades ahead nearly all of the increase in meat consumption will take place in the developing world.

Most nutritionists endorse the consumption of some meat and milk products (beginning with mother's milk) as a source of beneficial micronutrients such as iron, zinc, calcium, and vitamins A and B12. Most of these same micronutrients are also available from plant sources, but in a form less easily taken up by the human body. Animal products can be particularly valuable for children going through a critical phase of accelerated physical growth and brain development in the first two years of life, and also for women with higher iron requirements in their reproductive years. At the same time, excessive consumption of meat and animal products is associated with a number of poor health outcomes, including a variety of cancers, heart diseases, and stroke. In urban China between 1982 and 2002, when meat and dairy products in the average diet increased from 11 percent by weight up to 25 percent, the prevalence of diabetes, hypertension, heart disease, and stroke all increased sharply as well.

Some cultures discourage meat consumption for religious reasons. In India, where Hindus consider cows to be sacred, 31 percent of all citizens are vegetarians. In Ethiopia, Orthodox Christians fast from consuming meat and dairy foods for approximately 250 days of the year. Observant Jews and Muslims do not eat pork. Vegetarians are now 10 percent of the population in the UK (but only 2 percent in France). Roughly 5 percent of Americans are vegetarians, abstaining completely from meat, including poultry and seafood (but usually not eggs and dairy products), although some will eventually revert to a non-vegetarian diet. Vegans, who abstain from all animal products, are also a growing share of the population. Vegetarians and vegans together made up 10 percent of the US population in 2022, according to one online survey. Some become vegans or vegetarians because they dislike the way food animals are treated, or because they believe it is unethical to take the life of an animal for food. Some meat eaters have decided that the ethical issue is how well the animals are treated while alive, providing their death in the slaughterhouse is both unanticipated and virtually instantaneous.

Animal welfare and personal health concerns have recently given vegetarian and vegan diets a strong popular cachet. Film stars ranging from Brad Pitt and Woody Harrelson to Joaquin Phoenix have made it known that they are vegetarians, and in 2010 former president Bill Clinton followed his daughter's lead and adopted a vegan diet (after getting two stents on top of quadruple bypass surgery), explaining that he wanted to live to be a grandfather. NFL football star Tom Brady, the greatest quarterback of all time, has claimed to follow an "80 percent vegan" diet. Of course, committed vegans would insist on 100 percent.

Is a vegetarian diet healthier?

Dietary health requires a balance of nutrients, and for most people meat is a convenient part of this balance, but it is not strictly necessary. The Mayo Clinic confirms that even for growing children and adolescents vegetarian diets can be safe and healthy. Getting protein is not a problem, since vegetarians who are not vegans can get animal protein from milk and eggs, and even vegans can get abundant protein from beans, legumes, and nuts. Calcium is not a problem for vegetarians who consume dairy products, and vegans can get calcium from green vegetables or from products fortified with calcium, such as soymilks, cereals, and juices. Vegans must take special care to get vitamins D and B12, and the latter in particular may require seeking out fortified foods or supplements.

It is more convenient to secure the needed balance of nutrients from less restrictive non-vegetarian diets, but many who do will lapse into imbalances of other kinds. Non-vegetarian diets too often include inadequate helpings of fruits and vegetables, too much red meat, too many processed meats like bacon, sausage, and salami (containing risk-inducing nitrites as preservatives), and too many overcooked charred meats that carry cancer risks. When it comes to health, what matters most about meat is the quantity consumed and the way it was processed or cooked, not the fact that it is meat. One 2005 study from the German Cancer Research Center compared health-conscious meat eaters to vegetarians and found no difference in mortality rates.

In some societies, purely vegetarian diets are simply not an option. On drylands in Africa where there is not enough water for vegetable crops, many communities could not be sustained without cattle, sheep, and goats, which are ruminant animals with an extra stomach, allowing them to thrive on grasses that people cannot digest, converting those grasses into meat and milk for people. Likewise in arctic regions, human societies could not survive if they did not eat meat from fish and animals. Even in agricultural societies where producing vegetable food is an option, the sale of meat or milk from animals can be an essential household income source, especially for women and those who lack access to cropland.

If people in rich countries ate less meat, would hunger be reduced in poor countries?

Yes, but only by a small amount. If meat consumption declined, international meat and animal feed prices would also decline, but this would matter little for the vast proportion of hungry people, because they do not consume much that comes from the world market, particularly not meat or the grains fed to animals. What these poor people need is more income, to purchase rice, white maize, sorghum, millet, yams, cassava, or banana in their own local markets, not a lower international price for meat or animal feed. The effects of lower meat consumption in rich countries would mostly be confined to those same rich countries. Fewer cattle would be grazed on rangelands in Texas or Australia, but many of these lands are too dry for growing crops so they would simply go unused. Less corn and soy would be produced for animal feed, and this would free up some land for wheat and rice production, but the impact on international wheat and rice prices would be small.

The International Food Policy Research Institute has used a computer model of global agricultural markets to estimate the reduction in hunger that would result from a 50 percent reduction in per capita meat consumption in all high-income countries, from current levels. Under this extremely unlikely scenario, there would be 700,000 fewer chronically malnourished children in the developing world by the year 2030, compared to a "business as usual" scenario. This seems to be a measurable gain, but it is very small relative to the size of the problem. Under the "business as usual" scenario, there would be 134 million cases of child malnutrition in 2030, so the payoff from a 50 percent cut in meat consumption in rich countries is only a one-half of 1 percent reduction in child hunger. Reducing meat consumption in rich countries remains an excellent idea for the purpose of improving health and moderating environmental damage in those same rich countries, but not for getting more food to the hungry.

Will imitation meat replace the real thing?

One suggested pathway for reducing animal product consumption is substitution, with plant-based or cell-grown products that simulate the look and taste of meat while being "animal free." In the United States these products gained a foothold during the COVID-19 pandemic, when total refrigerated plant-based imitation meat sales increased 75 percent between 2019 and 2020. This growth slowed in 2022, however, and the Beyond Meat company reduced its workforce by 20 percent.

Today's imitation products are significantly more expensive than real ground beef; they are little better for dietary health; and taste differences remain; but they alleviate animal welfare concerns and they are dramatically better for the environment. The carbon footprint of an Impossible Burger is almost 90 percent smaller than that of a real beef burger. This plant-based alternative is 87 percent less dependent on water, and 96 percent less dependent on land.

Market shares for plant-based meats have remained small, making up just 2.7 percent of all US retail packaged "meat" sales in 2020. Sales of plant-based "milk" made from almonds, rice, or coconut made up 15 percent of all retail sales in the milk category. All plant-based imitation foods together generated $7 billion in US retail sales in 2020, which was a bit more than total retail sales for baked goods.

While plant-based meat substitutes are becoming established, a second approach to alternative meats—culturing real animal cells outside of living animals—has moved more slowly. In the United States, the FDA did not give regulatory approval to a cell-grown product until November 2022, when it finally approved chicken nuggets from a California company, Upside Foods. Singapore had earlier granted a similar regulatory approval in 2020.

Assuming the retail price of plant-based imitation meat continues to fall, some consumers will substitute for the real thing, and the production of real meat will then fall as well, but possibly not by much. According to one market model simulation, a 10 percent fall in the retail price of plant-based imitation meat might, by itself, result in only a 0.15 percent fall in the number of domestic cattle slaughtered. To get a steeper fall, the willingness of consumers to pay for substitutes will have to increase. The best solution to this problem will be the development of more delicious substitutes, and a wider variety of products beyond just ground beef and chicken nuggets. Rather than wait for market forces to deliver improved substitutes, governments viewing such products as a win for the environment might direct more public money toward R&D.

One surprising impediment to this important public policy opportunity has been a cool response to animal-free products from longtime critics of the livestock industry. Mark Bittman, a prominent food writer who once accused the livestock industry of "torturing billions of animals," is nonetheless critical of imitation meats because they are manufactured and inauthentic: "If you're combining a bunch of powders and turning it into something that looks like meat, I'm not sure you're doing anybody any good. I don't think it moves people in the direction of real food—which is the ultimate goal." For other food movement leaders, the fact that plant-based substitutes are heavily processed is reason enough to object. Brian Niccole, CEO of Chipotle, has said he won't serve plant-based meats "because of the processing," and Whole Foods CEO John Mackey, despite being a vegan himself, had a similar reaction: "If you look at the ingredients, they are super, highly processed foods."

What are CAFOs?

Concentrated animal feeding operations, called CAFOs, are highly specialized industrial-scale facilities where large numbers of animals are kept in confinement for poultry, egg, pork, or dairy production. In wealthy countries, led by the United States, these systems have largely replaced the pasture and barnyard-style livestock systems earlier common on small, diversified farms. CAFOs are a proven way to deliver higher volumes of standardized animal products to consumers at a much lower market price, mostly because they save on labor and land costs, yet they have generated strong opposition from advocates for animal welfare, public health, and environmental protection.

In the United States, CAFOs spread first to the egg and poultry sector in the 1950s, then to the swine and dairy sector in the 1970s and 1980s. Beef cattle still spend most of their lives grazing on pasture, but are fattened for the last four to six months in a confined feedlot. CAFOs are defined by the Environmental Protection Agency (EPA) according to the number of animals they house. If an animal feeding operation has more than 700 mature dairy cattle, more than 1,000 cattle, or more than 30,000 laying hens or broiler chickens, it is considered a "large" CAFO and is automatically subject to EPA regulation under the Clean Water Act. CAFOs have spread internationally and are now widely used in Europe, and have also become prevalent in China, Thailand, and Vietnam, driven by rapidly rising consumer demand for meat, poultry, and eggs. The UN Food and Agriculture Organization (FAO) has estimated that 80 percent of all growth in livestock production around the world now takes place within "industrial" CAFO-style systems.

Are CAFOs bad for animal welfare?

CAFOs manage farm animals under highly regulated conditions, typically in crowded confinement. Automated feed delivery and waste removal replace grazing and foraging, eliminating many traditional husbandry practices performed by human labor. This approach reduces land, labor, and facilities costs per unit of meat or milk produced, but even within the best maintained facilities, the impacts on animal welfare are problematic. The animals may face fewer risks linked to weather exposure, zoonotic diseases, and wild predators, and in some instances less harm from social conflict with each other, but they will be denied opportunities to engage in numerous instinctive behaviors—such as walking, perching, wing-flapping, or foraging—that have long been central to their daily routines. For example, in CAFOs pregnant sows weighing 400 pounds may be confined to iron "gestation crates" 7 feet long and 22 inches wide, in which they are unable to turn around. They will be on slatted floors that make cleanup easier, but this will leave them with no bedding and nothing to root around in.

In 2005, the American Veterinary Medical Association—which has close ties to the livestock industry—convened a task force to determine whether sows were harmed by this kind of confinement, and found that the research was mixed. Confinement in crates can protect low-status sows from being bitten by high-status sows, but the welfare of all will suffer if the animals are unable to turn around. Animal welfare advocates believe the CAFO model is harmful not only to sows in crates but also to egg-laying hens in small "battery" cages. In 2011, an agricultural economist at Oklahoma State University used a mathematical welfare model for egg-laying hens plus his own judgments to conclude that hens in small cages have a negative welfare score and would thus be "better off euthanized."

The Humane Society of the United States (HSUS) and other advocacy groups, such as People for Ethical Treatment of Animals (PETA), have waged campaigns to restrict or even eliminate the use of crates and cages. Sometimes these campaigns take the form of state-by-state ballot issues placed before voters, and increasingly they have been successful. Arizona, California, Colorado, Florida, Maine, Massachusetts, Michigan, Ohio, and Rhode Island have banned the use of sow gestation crates. California, Massachusetts, Michigan, Ohio, Oregon, and Washington have nixed battery cages for hens. Meanwhile, in response to consumer demands, corporate meat buyers have also started demanding changes. More than 60 companies—including McDonald's, Burger King, Oscar Mayer, Costco, and Kroger—have now promised only to buy and sell crate-free pork. Whole Foods Market and Chipotle met that goal by 2016.

In the United States, CAFOs are regulated for human health and safety, and for environmental protection, but until recently there have been few laws governing the welfare of the animals, beyond those that apply to humane transport and slaughter. The United States does have laws to protect companion animal welfare (the Animal Welfare Act of 1966), but farm animals were excluded, and between 1985 and 1995, to make things worse, at least 18 states passed laws explicitly exempting agriculture from existing animal cruelty laws. Other countries have embraced higher standards. In 1991, the UK government required pig farmers to have their animals in pens rather than crates by 1999. Pig-producing nations in the European Union (EU) were told to have their sows in pens rather than crates by 2013. These reforms have been surprisingly affordable. In 2015, after the swine rules came into effect, one study found that total carcass-weight production costs in the EU averaged 19 percent higher than in Canada, and 38 percent higher than in the United States, but these differences mostly reflected higher feed and labor costs in Europe, not the added cost of more spacious housing under the new regulations. In countries like the Netherlands, housing makes up only a little more than one-tenth of total production costs. Some countries like Germany have gone much farther, by introducing in 2003 a requirement that pigs have access to sunlight, toys for amusement, and at least 20 seconds of personal contact with the farmer every day. Skeptics suspect such regulations will prove difficult to enforce.

Tighter animal welfare regulations will increase costs, but the industry can adjust if granted a transition period, and most proposed reforms will be easily affordable for consumers. When the McDonald's Corporation began insisting on larger cages for egg-laying hens, the resulting increase in cost to consumers was calculated at only about 1 penny per egg.

What else generates opposition to CAFOs?

Critics of CAFOs point to several concerns beyond the welfare of the animals. One worry, partly inspired by the COVID-19 pandemic, is the spread of disease from the crowding together of large numbers of animals, all with similar genetics. On the other hand, bringing the animals indoors in biosecure buildings actually reduces their exposure to the many parasites and pathogens found in open environments. Tapeworm parasites were not eliminated from the meat supply in Europe and North America until small-scale pig rearing was replaced by confinement production. Likewise the incidence of trichinosis in the United States declined from 400 clinical cases annually to only 60 cases between the 1940s and the 1980s, primarily through a better control of infections offered by indoor pig farming. In a similar way, the pathogen *T. gondii* was found in one out of five marketed hogs in the 1980s, but that prevalence has now been reduced by over 90 percent. Dr. Rodney Baker, a former president of the American Association of Swine Veterinarians, asserts, "By bringing the animals indoors and creating biosecurity, we've truly eliminated about 15 diseases and parasites we had back to the 1980s."

The use of antibiotics in livestock feed to promote weight gain is another concern, since it creates a human health risk by speeding the emergence of resistant bacterial strains. This is a legitimate concern in the United States. The livestock industry claims that only one-third of the antibiotics it employs are used in human medicine, but little data have been shared on how specific drugs are administered, to which animals, and why. After the FDA began monitoring the presence of antibiotic-resistant bacteria in retail meat in 1996, through a National Antimicrobial Resistance Monitoring System (NARMS), a report released in 2013 indicated that over the previous decade ampicillin resistance in retail chickens had increased from 17 percent to 40 percent. Finally, in 2012, a federal district court judge in New York ordered the FDA to ban the use of low-dose penicillin and two forms of tetracycline for weight gain purposes, so FDA initiated a three-year phase-out of antibiotic use on livestock for growth promotion purposes, and it phased in a requirement for veterinary oversight of antibiotic use.

Experience in the EU shows that antibiotic use in CAFOs can be reduced affordably. The bloc banned the use of antimicrobials to promote weight gain in 2006, and in January 2022 it specified that these drugs can no longer be given preventatively en masse, or used to compensate for overcrowding. Because overcrowding is also better regulated in Europe, these measures had only a small impact on meat production. Following the 2006 ban in the Netherlands, pig inventories remained essentially unchanged even as sales of antimicrobials fell by two-thirds.

A third concern is microbial contamination in meat. This can be a serious health threat, but the contamination is usually introduced in the slaughterhouse after the animal has left the CAFO, or in the consumer's own kitchen, and the frequency of contamination in the United States has been greatly reduced in any case. For fresh ground beef, the USDA found that the presence of a particularly dangerous strain of *E. coli*, 0157:H7 declined by 63 percent after 2000, down to only one-third of 1 percent. Salmonella on chicken declined by 21 percent, and on fresh pork by 63 percent. *Listeria monocytogenes* declined by 74 percent on ready-to-eat meat and poultry products.

Popular films such as *Food, Inc.* have claimed that cattle fed on corn in feedlots, rather than raised exclusively on pasture, will be more prone to grow *E. coli* O157:H7 in their digestive system, increasing the likelihood of meat contamination during slaughter and processing. Grass-fed beef is certainly more nutritious than feed-lot beef, because it has less fat, more vitamin A and E, and more omega-3 fatty acids, but there is no convincing scientific evidence that it is any less prone to O157:H7. For example, one study published in *Applied & Environmental Microbiology* in 2009 concluded, "Our study found similar prevalences of *E. coli* O157:H7 in the feces of organically and naturally raised beef cattle [on grass], and our prevalence estimates for cattle from these types of production systems are similar to those reported previously for conventionally raised feedlot cattle."

Strong opposition to CAFOs also emerges on environmental grounds. Concentrating hundreds or even thousands
of animals in a confined space creates a concentrated threat to
local air and water quality from the urine and manure of the
animals. The resulting environmental harms may include excess nutrients in water (particularly nitrogen and phosphorus),
which in turn can contribute to low levels of dissolved oxygen,
leading to fish kills. Decomposing organic matter can also contribute to toxic algal blooms. CAFO systems attempt to con-
fine the animal waste within onsite "lagoons," to be recycled
later in a safe and controlled manner, but lagoon leakage can
introduce pathogens into local drinking water. The EPA has
calculated that states with high concentrations of CAFOs experience on average 20 to 30 serious water quality problems per
year. Dust and odors can lead to worker illness and respiratory
problems for those living downwind from CAFOs.

In the United States, CAFOs have been regulated since
1972 under the Clean Water Act as "point sources" of pollution. A permit program sets effluent limit guidelines, and the
guidelines were revised in 2003 to require that all permitted
CAFOs develop nutrient management plans, but the guidelines
were revised again in 2008 to require permits only for those
CAFOs planning to discharge waste, a major loophole since
the most environmentally damaging discharges are usually
unplanned. In 1995, an eight-acre hog-waste lagoon in North
Carolina burst, spilling 25 million gallons of manure into the
New River, killing about 10 million fish and closing 364,000
acres of coastal wetlands to shellfishing. Two years later, a new
state law was passed placing a moratorium on new construction of hog farms with more than 250 animals. Then, when
Hurricane Floyd hit North Carolina in 1999, at least five more
manure lagoons burst and approximately 47 lagoons were
completely flooded.

Ponds and streams in rural America have always been
polluted by animal waste, but usually in a widely dispersed
pattern. Thanks to the growth of CAFOs, more than half of all

the hogs raised in the United States are concentrated in just three states: Iowa, North Carolina, and Minnesota. This can generate a far more concentrated pollution risk for nearby communities.

Improved methods are becoming available to manage waste from CAFOs, and also methane emissions. Anaerobic digesters that trap methane from covered waste lagoons are coming into wider use on large dairy farms. Farmers can then sell the gas into pipelines to fuel vehicles powered by renewable natural gas (RNG). In 2021 there were 185 digesters either functioning or under construction to service 194 dairies in California alone. Compared to gasoline vehicles, RNG cars burn 49 percent less carbon.

Another forward-looking approach is to give feed additives to cattle that reduce the methane produced in their digestive system. In February 2022, the Dutch company DSM received preliminary approval in the EU for an additive named Bovaer that suppresses the triggering enzyme for methane in the cow's rumen. A quarter teaspoon of Bovaer per cow per day reduces enteric methane emissions by 30 percent for dairy cows, and as much as 90 percent for beef cattle, with no adverse health consequences.

How important are fish as a source of food?

Fish and fishery products are a valuable source of both protein and essential micronutrients. Globally, protein consumption from fish exceeds that from poultry or pork, and it is more than twice as high as animal protein consumption from beef and veal. Fish are central to traditional diets in many cultures, particularly in Asia. Fish consumption is lowest in Africa, with only 10 kilograms per person per year. In the United States and Europe it is more than 20 kilograms per person, in China it is nearly 40 kilograms per capita, and in Japan more than 40 kilograms. More than two-thirds of all fish consumption takes place in Asia.

Growth in global fish consumption has been high, averaging 3.2 percent annually over the past half century. Fish used for food can either be from inland freshwater or from ocean saltwater, and may be either captured or farmed. People eat not only finfish but many other water species as well, including large quantities of crustaceans such as crab; mollusks such as clams, mussels, and squid; plus various other aquatic animals such as sea urchins. Traditionally, most fish consumption has been satisfied through capture (popular author Paul Greenberg has labeled fish "the last wild food"), but now more than half the global supply comes from fish farming, referred to as aquaculture. Current moves toward farming fish are not so different from the first human efforts to domesticate meat animals and crops 10,000 years ago.

Are wild fisheries collapsing?

The total marine (ocean) capture of fish peaked in 1996 at 86 million tons. It briefly declined but has now stabilized at roughly 80 million tons, except for a dip in 2020 due to COVID-19 lockdowns. Inland fish capture has also been stable recently, at about 12 million tons, so wild fisheries are not "collapsing." Globally, 66 percent of monitored fisheries are at biologically sustainable levels while producing 78.7 percent of consumed seafood. The 34 percent of fisheries that are producing below 80 percent of sustainable levels (the share that are "overfished") produce 22.3 percent of seafood. Overfishing can put dangerous stress on a vast natural ecology, threatening more than just human welfare or food security.

The overexploitation of marine fisheries has technological, economic, and political origins. The technology for finding and catching fish has steadily improved. Long-Range Navigation (LORAN), Global Positioning Systems (GPS), and Geographic Information Systems (GIS) allow vessels today to pinpoint the most productive fishing grounds, and recent refinements to sonar technology even allow fishers to more quickly find distinct species of fish. To locate swordfish and tuna, aircraft are deployed with infrared sensors that detect subtle changes in the surface temperature of the ocean. Airborne electronic image intensifiers also can be used to detect the light given off at night by some marine algae when disturbed by passing schools of fish.

The economic driver for overexploitation is global income growth, particularly in Asia. In China, where consumers for centuries have considered fish beneficial to the brain, income growth has fueled high demand. Between 1990 and 2019, prior to a dip during COVID-19, per capita fish consumption in China increased at an average annual rate of 6 percent, reaching nearly 40 kilograms. Fortunately, a growing share of China's appetite for fish is now satisfied through aquaculture; China by itself in 2018–2020 was the site of 57 percent of all global aquaculture production. Regionally, China and the rest of Asia will likely be home to 88 percent of the world's aquaculture production by 2030.

The political drivers for overfishing are more subtle. National governments have come to recognize the importance of making fishing sustainable, and under the UN Convention on the Law of the Sea they terminated open access to coastal fisheries by claiming waters within 200 miles of their shores as an exclusive economic zone (EEZ). In these waters off the coast of the United States, stocks are now better protected thanks to a 1996 law, the Magnuson-Stevens Fishery Conservation and Management Act, that set targets for rebuilding each species. As of 2013, 21 of 44 species had met the rebuilding target, and 7 others had made significant progress, increasing their populations by at least 25 percent. As of 2020, annual catch limits were being enforced for approximately 90 percent of all stocks. When catch limit overages occur, the National Oceanic and Atmospheric Administration in the Department of Commerce takes steps to ensure they don't continue.

Fish that migrate beyond an EEZ remain at serious risk of overexploitation. In the open ocean, restricting the catch requires international cooperation, and this has not yet been forthcoming. In 2010 international concern for bluefin tuna stocks, which had declined by 75 percent, triggered a proposal to ban international trade in bluefin tuna under the Convention on International Trade in Endangered Species (CITES), but the measure was blocked by states with a strong commercial interest in the catch. Japan, which imports 80 percent of Atlantic bluefin, led the opposition, but more than 70 other countries opposed the trade ban as well. Trade bans on fish are potentially powerful instruments, since 37 percent of fishery production enters international commerce, with the EU by itself taking more than 40 percent of all global imports, followed by the United States, China, and Japan. Both the United States and Japan depend on imports for more than half of their domestic consumption.

Sustainable stocks management is also frustrated by fishing activities that are illegal, unreported, and unregulated, known as IUU. Many developing countries lack the physical or technical capacity to patrol their EEZ, and in some cases government officials in those countries are easily bribed into giving permits to those who overfish. Most regional fisheries are nominally governed by regional fishery bodies (RFBs), but these organizations depend too much on voluntary compliance by member governments, many of whom are unwilling or unable to exercise control. To supplement these RFBs, the United States and the EU have been cooperating bilaterally since 2011, looking for better ways to keep IUU fish off the world market.

Is fish farming a solution?

Fish can be raised in tanks and ponds, and even in oceans, lakes, and rivers with the aid of cages or nets. Fully "farmed" fish are those hatched from eggs within the aquaculture facility and confined for their entire life cycle, whereas "ranched" fish spend part of their lives in the wild. Some will be hatched and released, then caught when they return (like ranched salmon), while others will be caught in the wild as juveniles, then fed in confinement until they reach market weight (like ranched bluefin tuna).

The global aquaculture industry is growing rapidly, both in fresh and saltwater. Between the decade that began in 1986 and calendar year 2018, total production from aquaculture, both inland and marine, increased from 14.9 million tons up to 82.1 million tons. This rapid growth is expected to continue in India, Indonesia, Vietnam, and Thailand as well as in China. The favored species will include tilapia, shrimps and prawns, and carp, which have been farmed in Chinese ponds for centuries. Two-thirds of all aquaculture species must be provided with feed, which is an increasingly significant feature of the industry.

Small scale, pond-based inland aquaculture can provide both food and income to poor rural communities. As recently as 1990, when rice consumption dominated diets in Bangladesh, annual per capita fish consumption was only 10 kilograms, and 51 percent of children under age five were stunted. Then, between 1990 and 2012 production from fish farming tripled. By 2018 per capita fish consumption had more than doubled, and the rate of child stunting had fallen to 31 percent.

The rapid growth of aquaculture has relieved some commercial pressure on wild fisheries, but the industry nonetheless remains controversial, often because of unsolved technical problems. Disease outbreaks have affected farmed Atlantic salmon in Chile, oysters in Europe, and marine shrimp in Asia, South America, and Africa. In 2011, a disease outbreak nearly wiped out marine shrimp farming in Mozambique.

In other cases, interactions between farmed and wild species are a concern. When wild Atlantic salmon collapsed as a commercial fishery in the 1960s, it was replaced by highly affordable farmed Atlantic salmon, but the farmed fish are often grown along wild salmon migration routes, posing risks such as food-borne diseases and parasites, and wastes that create a pollution problem. A larger concern for carnivorous fish such as salmon and tuna is the toll taken on wild fish caught as forage, including herring and sardines. It requires 5–15 pounds of wild fish to grow a single pound of Atlantic bluefin tuna in a net pen, and overharvesting forage fish could bring damage to multiple commercial species.

In the United States, the fish farming industry is politically weak compared to crop and livestock producers, partly because it is so new and nontraditional. America has no national fish farming heritage to invoke, there is no established cabinet agency to support fish farming, and no tradition of property rights for fish farmers. In addition, there is often strong local opposition from environmentalists and from residential and recreational users of water resources. Similar political and institutional patterns are visible in much of Europe. For these reasons, the industry is likely to continue to expand most rapidly in the developing countries of Asia, and American and European consumers will become increasingly dependent on imports of farmed fish from abroad.

11

AGRIBUSINESS, FOOD COMPANIES, SUPERMARKETS, AND FAST FOOD

What does the word "agribusiness" mean?

The term "agribusiness" was coined in 1957 by two professors at the Harvard Business School, Ray Goldberg and John H. Davis, in recognition of an important change then taking place in the American agricultural sector. The "on-farm" part of America's food economy was shrinking relative to input supply industries upstream (seed, farm chemical, and machinery suppliers) and also relative to food storage, transport, processing, manufacturing, packaging, marketing, retail, and food service industries downstream. Since farms had become just one part of a longer and more industrialized food value chain, it made sense to begin referring to the chain as a single integrated entity: agribusiness.

The new term stuck, a *Journal of Agribusiness* was founded, and soon after, more than 100 institutions of higher education in the United States began offering formal degrees in agribusiness. In 1990, the International Food and Agribusiness Management Association (IAMA) was founded as a worldwide networking organization and a bridge among multinational agribusiness companies, researchers, educators, and government officials.

Why is agribusiness controversial?

Among those who work within most food and farm industries, the word "agribusiness" is used in a descriptive, nonjudgmental way; the term even carries a flattering connotation of modernity. Yet for critics outside the sector, the term carries negative connotations. It is deployed to suggest that traditional and trustworthy family farmers have been replaced by powerful profit-driven corporations not accountable for the damage they do to rural communities, human health, and the environment.

Strong critiques of American agribusiness date from 1973, when a Texas populist named Jim Hightower published a book titled *Hard Tomatoes, Hard Times*. Hightower argued that corporate power now dominated not only farming but also the US Department of Agriculture and even the nation's agricultural universities, leading to a more rapid demise of small farms, displacing farmworkers and bringing us unhealthy food. Agribusiness firms were also a target of journalist Eric Schlosser's widely popular 1999 book *Fast Food Nation: The Dark Side of the All-American Meal*. More recently, in 2009, a popular film titled *Food, Inc.* asserted that "our nation's food supply is now controlled by a handful of corporations that often put profit ahead of consumer health, the livelihood of the American farmer, the safety of workers and our own environment." In 2022, Cory Booker (D-NJ) introduced a Food and Agribusiness Merger Moratorium and Antitrust Review Act into the Senate, to fight against economic concentration in the food sector by placing a moratorium on certain acquisitions between large agricultural and retail-related businesses.

Over the years the critics have identified favorite corporate villains along every separate link in the value chain. Chemical companies and multinational seed companies have tended to attract the greatest criticism, and because the St. Louis–based Monsanto Company (acquired in 2018 by Bayer, a German company) was both a chemical company (selling herbicides) and a multinational biotechnology company (developing and patenting genetically engineered crop seeds), it became the most vilified of all. Downstream from farms, among firms that ship and handle farm commodities, a large company from Minneapolis named Cargill was earlier a favorite target, both for its secrecy as a privately held firm and for its alleged market power. Within the meat sector, Tyson Foods, Inc., of Springdale, Arkansas, the world's largest processor and marketer of chicken, beef, and pork, is often depicted as an enemy of small family farmers and a threat to the environment. In the packaged food sector, ConAgra Foods, Inc., of Omaha, Nebraska, is said to damage consumer health by marketing heavily processed and chemical-laden foods such as frozen dinners, Slim Jims, and Reddi-wip. Big manufacturers of sugar-sweetened beverages are also a target. Finally, at the retail and food service end, Walmart has been accused of mistreating workers and McDonald's and Burger King are accused of addicting children to unhealthy burgers, fries, and sweetened drinks.

In 2019, before the COVID-19 pandemic, restaurants in America delivered $864 billion worth of meals and service to their customers, more than twice the total value of all US farm sales that year, so the American economy now generates much more money *serving* food than it does growing food. The USDA calculated in 2017 that only 7.8 percent of the average food consumer's dollar could be traced to on-farm and upstream activities; 17.3 percent was attributable to processing and packaging by food manufacturing companies, 12.6 percent to food retailers, and 36.7 percent to food service.

Food industries have long been an inviting target for populist attack. In 1906, a muckraking novel by Upton Sinclair, titled *The Jungle*, exposed disgraceful working conditions in Chicago's meatpacking industry. Like many critics of agribusiness today, Sinclair was motivated by his personal suspicion of private corporations in general, and he used the emotive issue of food to dramatize this larger suspicion. The book caused a sensation, but most readers skipped over the labor rights message and focused instead on a worry that industrial meat products might not be safe to eat. Sinclair's book led directly to passage of the Meat Inspection Act and the Pure Food and Drug Act of 1906 and to the creation of a national Food and Drug Administration (FDA).

Do agribusiness firms control farmers?

Farmers in America have always worried about the market power of non-farmers. Historically, they worried most about bankers, railroads, and grain traders; today, they worry more about concentration in the seed industry and in the meatpacking industry, where the market power of private companies vis-à-vis farmers has recently increased.

A fear of industry concentration in the international seed sector has arisen since the 1990s, following a proliferation of patent claims on genetically engineered seeds, accompanied by a frenzy of corporate mergers and acquisitions. Between 1985 and 2009, annual sales in global seed markets increased from $18 billion to about $44 billion, and by 2008 the Monsanto Company and its subsidiaries owned more than 400 separate plant technology patents and claimed more than 20 percent of the global proprietary seed market. The top five companies had 54 percent. New alarm bells went off in 2018 when Monsanto was purchased (for $63 billion) by the German conglomerate Bayer. To satisfy antitrust lawyers in the Justice Department, Bayer had to sell off $9 billion worth of assets. In the end, Bayer paid a big price for this acquisition, because along with Monsanto's crop science capabilities, it acquired the legal liabilities associated with lawsuits from cancer victims claiming damages from a Monsanto herbicide with the trade name Roundup.

In the developing world, seed industry concentration will have limited reach because most countries still do not allow seeds to be patented, and the vast majority do not even allow genetically engineered seeds to be planted. In addition, commercial seed markets provide only one part of the world's total seed supply. Many farmers in poor countries, and quite a few in rich countries as well, do not buy any seeds at all on a regular basis, instead planting the seeds they save from their own harvest.

Seed companies like Monsanto/Bayer have enforced their patent claims in part through contracts with farmers called stewardship agreements, where farmers agree not to save and replant the patented seeds after harvest. The companies are also willing to go to court. According to one tally done by the Center for Food Safety in 2013, Monsanto had filed more than 140 patent infringement lawsuits over the years, collecting a total of $24 million in recorded judgments. This did represent a new element of corporate control over farmers, but economic studies of the corn and cottonseed industries showed that the patented seeds brought cost-reducing benefits to farmers that significantly outweighed any disadvantage posed by the patent claims or from greater corporate concentration. Farmers buy these seeds because the traits help them cut production costs significantly. When patent-owning companies set their prices too high, as in the case of Monsanto's bungled introduction of a new SmartStax corn variety in 2010, farmers balk and start buying seed from another company (in this case, from an Iowa-based rival, DuPont Pioneer). In 2009, DuPont Pioneer pressed the Obama administration to initiate antitrust action against Monsanto, but a multiyear Justice Department investigation into Monsanto was closed in 2012, without any action taken.

Market concentration in the seed sector is to some extent an artifact of the stigmatizing political attacks leveled against genetically engineered seeds that dried up European investment in this technology, leaving US companies like Monsanto with few international competitors. In retrospect, more government research money could have been used to develop this new seed technology in the public sector without patent restrictions, but Congress had cut back on such funding, giving private companies greater space to claim dominance.

The American meat processing sector has also become highly concentrated in recent decades. In 1977, the four largest beef packing firms—Cargill, Tyson Foods, JBS, and National Beef Packing—had 25 percent of the market; today they have 82 percent. The four largest firms in pork and poultry also control a majority of the market in those sectors. In 2021 the Biden administration began investigations to determine if this degree of market concentration had allowed the firms to pay lower prices to producers while charging higher prices to consumers. Tyson agreed in 2021 to pay $221.5 million to settle accusations of conspiring to inflate chicken prices, and in 2022 JBS agreed to pay $52.5 million to settle a lawsuit brought by grocery stores and wholesalers, which accused the big four meatpackers of conspiring to drive up beef prices.

Companies such as Tyson Foods work with thousands of individual "contract chicken growers" who provide their own land and construct their own sheds to raise the chickens, while the company owns the chickens and provides all the feed. The growers who work for agribusiness firms under this sort of contract, as well as those still struggling to survive as independents, have reason to fear that the companies will use their market power to gain a disproportionate advantage. In the 1990s, America's hog slaughter industry also moved toward greater vertical integration and concentration, a move that left even the remaining independent producers with less market control.

Outside of the biotech seed sector and the livestock sector, corporations do not yet have significant market power over farmers. The largest portion of all basic crop production in the United States now comes from very large farms, but more than 96 percent of farms and ranches are still family owned. Many are corporations, but with more than half of the voting stock held by family members. Non-family corporations account for only 6 percent of all farm sales. As for control from downstream crop purchasing companies, competitive markets tend to prevail here as well, in part because concentration among the purchasing companies is offset by the counter-vailing power of farmer-controlled marketing cooperatives, which can be formed legally under America's federal mar-keting order system.

It is a stretch to imagine, as some do, that international corporations control the lives of poor farmers in the devel-oping world. Most poor farmers in Africa do not make any purchases of seeds at all (they save seeds from the previous season's crop), and they make only minimal purchases of fertilizers and pesticides. When they market a portion of their crop, it is usually to local buyers or to government-regulated marketing boards, rather than to vertically integrated agribusi-ness firms. Private international agribusiness companies pay little attention to most small farmers in Africa, because those farmers lack the productivity to be good suppliers along with the purchasing power needed to be good customers. In Africa, only 2 percent of all investment in agricultural research comes from private firms. There is little danger that international investors will control poor farmers in Africa; the bigger risk is that they will continue to ignore them.

Do food companies and supermarkets control consumers?

Food manufacturing and retailing have also undergone market concentration, but this is not their most important source of influence over consumers. A 2021 investigation by industry critics found that four firms or fewer controlled at least 50 per-cent of the market for 79 percent of the groceries Americans buy. For almost a third of individual shopping items, the top firms controlled at least 75 percent of the market share. For example, PepsiCo controlled 88 percent of the dip market (it owns five of the most popular brands including Tostitos, Lay's and Fritos). Ninety-three percent of the sodas we drink are owned by just three companies. The same goes for 73 percent of the breakfast cereals we eat.

Critics suspect that food manufacturing companies and retail supermarket chains exploit their concentrated market power to raise the cost of food to consumers, and careful studies by economists show that concentration in the food manufacturing sector does raise costs to consumers, but only by a small percentage. Bruce Gardner, a leading American agricultural economist, calculated that in the 1990s only about 2 percent of the consumer's final marketing bill went to pay for "excess profits" due to imperfect market competition. With respect to supermarkets, studies show that retailing has also become more concentrated, and in cities with fewer competing stores consumer food prices are indeed higher. Yet the rate of profit in the retail food industry overall, measured per dollar of sales, has not increased over time, thanks to efficiencies from larger store size that are passed on to consumers. Instead of controlling consumers, modern supermarkets compete with each other to attract customers by attempting to offer an ever-growing array of popular and affordable food purchase options.

Some food companies have clearly held near-monopoly positions for individual food products. For example, General Foods has enjoyed nearly 90 percent of the market in Jell-O-like products. Yet there is no convincing evidence that the company's profits from Jell-O have been higher than for products such as peanut butter, where there is much more competition. If profits begin moving up, competitors will move in, as in the case of the creatively blended ice cream sold by Ben & Jerry's, which became so successful that it quickly inspired competing alternative brands. The American food industry had more than 31,000 food and beverage processing companies in 2017, with many emerging or going out of business every year. The new companies that do well are often acquired by the big conglomerates capable of bringing these successful brands to a mass customer base, but it is popularity with consumers, not corporate control, that drives this outcome.

In one respect, however, food companies have learned to control consumer choice. As noted in Chapter 7, food companies—and also restaurant chains—have designed many of their offerings to be virtually addictive.

Are supermarkets spreading into developing countries?

The supermarkets that are pervasive in rich countries have spread rapidly into the developing world, bringing more choices for consumers but also market disruptions for competing retailers and local food producers.

Supermarkets tend to spring up naturally wherever people get increased income, buy refrigerators and private automobiles, and wherever women have entered the workforce. North America, Europe, and Japan have fit this profile for decades, and in the United States today 92 percent of retail food sales are made through supermarkets, rather than through smaller specialty stores or convenience markets. France opened its first supermarket in 1958, and now two-thirds of national food retail sales are made in supermarkets. More noteworthy has been the recent and rapid spread of supermarkets into parts of the developing world despite the fact that affluence, auto ownership, and female workforce participation are not yet as pervasive.

In Latin America in the 1980s, only 10 percent of all food retail sales were made through supermarkets, but by 2000, that figure rose to 50–60 percent. Supermarkets took off five to seven years later in East Asia and Southeast Asia but then exhibited even faster growth. In Taiwan and South Korea, supermarket sales quickly gained a 63 percent share of all food sales. In China in 1991, there were no supermarkets at all, yet by 2001, the supermarket share in China's urban food markets was 48 percent. Supermarkets do not yet serve as many customers in South Asia or in Sub-Saharan Africa. For example, retail market shares in India and in Nigeria have struggled to reach 10 percent.

One key factor in the spread of supermarkets in poor countries has been electrification and the availability of home refrigerators, which make possible the purchase of fresh foods in larger quantity and on a less frequent basis. Second has been the opening of more national economies in the developing world to foreign direct investment, particularly since the 1990s. This gave established supermarket chains, such as Ahold, Carrefour, Tesco, and Walmart, opportunities to move quickly into the retail food markets of Latin America and Asia. Soon, three of every ten pesos spent on food in Mexico was being spent at a Walmart.

Local consumers generally benefit when supermarkets arrive, because they gain access to a wider variety of food purchase options that are offered at a higher standard for both food safety and cosmetic appearance, and usually at a lower cost. Some local farmers and local food wholesale and retail competitors will be threatened, however.

Small local farmers usually cannot provide the steady supply of top-quality fresh food that a multinational supermarket will require, because of small scale, inferior harvest methods, and a lack of post-harvest product protection. They are only able to offer smaller batches of lower-quality produce, so they tend to be bypassed by supermarket buyers, who source instead from modern-style specialty farms, including many created by foreign investors. These farms deliver contracted produce either to supermarkets directly or, more likely, to yet another new commercial institution, a "distribution center" that will serve as supplier to multiple local supermarkets. Systems of this kind bypass not just traditional local farms but also traditional urban wholesale markets. The rapid insertion of these exotic systems into food markets in the developing world has changed the diet of consumers (encouraging the consumption of more packaged foods, processed foods, and internationally branded imported foods) and also the market position of local food producers and wholesalers, because it keeps them away from the most affluent local customer base.

Is Walmart taking over food retailing in Africa and India?

Walmart is the world's largest retailer (of much more than just food). It is also the largest private employer in the world, with more than 10,000 stores in 24 different countries, under 46 different names. The company's data-mining capacity is second only to that of the Pentagon. Until recently, supermarkets like Walmart had a relatively small footprint both in Africa (where income growth is still lagging) and in India (mostly because the government of India did not allow foreign retailers majority ownership in "multi-brand" stores). Then, in 2011, Walmart decided to invest in Africa, purchasing for $2.4 billion a majority share in the South African retail chain Massmart, which operated 290 stores in 13 African countries. Walmart had earlier lost out in Asia to fast-moving rivals like Tesco and did not want this to happen in Africa.

Walmart's move into Africa did not go well. Massmart's growth stalled in the face of Africa's difficult regulatory environment, foreign exchange risks, and macroeconomic volatility. Burdened by debt and drowning in its lease obligations on commercial properties, Massmart was showing losses by 2019, and then in 2020 the COVID-19 pandemic created a shift toward online shopping that Massmart failed to take advantage of. But instead of giving up, as it had earlier in Germany, Walmart doubled down and in 2022 it unveiled a plan to take full control of Massmart. This was a risky decision because of the looming arrival in Africa of Amazon, a company that has outpaced Walmart in e-commerce inside the US market.

Walmart also struggled to get into India. In 2011 the Indian Cabinet approved a plan to permit foreign retailers majority ownership, but then pulled back for a year in the face of strong opposition from small traders and shopkeepers who feared they would be put out of business. But when India's economic growth began slowing in 2012, the government revived its plan to attract more foreign investment into the retail sector, and the president of Walmart's Indian unit responded by promising to come in as a good citizen, investing to help build the infrastructure that India needs to lower retail costs and reduce postharvest waste. Critics and opposition party leaders knew that Walmart was being investigated for earlier paying millions of dollars in bribes to local officials in Mexico when it expanded its operations there, and they warned that the same aggressive approach would be used to corrupt officials in India. Paying bribes ("speed money") to local officials is often the only way to make things happen in India, where in some states retail chains must secure 50 to 60 separate regulatory approvals before they can open a store. When India specified in 2013 that Walmart would have to source 30 percent of its products from local small-scale industries, the company gave up on its plans.

Are fast food restaurant chains spreading unhealthy eating habits worldwide?

Unhealthy eating styles are spreading globally. According to one estimate, by the decade that begins in 2040, people in today's low- and middle-income countries will be consuming as much unhealthy food as people today in rich countries. Increased consumption of packaged foods, snack foods, and soft drinks purchased from supermarkets will be part of this trend, but increased patronage at fast food ("quick-service") restaurant chains will contribute as well.

Quick-service chains went global in the 1980s and 1990s, moving into many countries alongside supermarkets and at an equally rapid rate. In 1990, South Korea had four McDonald's restaurants; five years later, it had 48. In the same short five-year period, China went from having one McDonald's restaurant to 62. Indonesia went from none to 38. Brazil went from 63 to 243. During this high-growth period, a new McDonald's restaurant was opening somewhere in the world every three hours. More than 60 percent of McDonald's global revenue now comes from outside the United States. Critics see this as an unfortunate imposition of bad food, plus America's garish commercial culture, onto vulnerable consumers in the developing world who are naively enthralled at becoming more "Western."

As usual, the picture is more complicated. In Asia and Africa quick-service "street food" for urbanites long predated the arrival of McDonald's restaurants. In Asia, takeaway stands selling salty fried foods have always been a not-so-healthy local option. In South Asia street foods abound, for example *panipuri*, which is fried bread with a spice and potato filling. In the Middle East, flatbread and falafel to go have long been found everywhere. In urban West Africa, ready-to-eat char-grilled meat sticks have long been popular. To some extent, Western fast foods are merely a replacement for these traditional local fast foods, many of which also fall short of providing a balanced diet.

On the issue of cultural imperialism, anthropologists who study the impact of fast food restaurants in developing countries have also reached more nuanced conclusions. In many East Asian settings, fast food restaurants did not directly replace traditional cuisine. They were often just a place to go for a snack between meals, or to socialize with friends after school. Asian customers saw fast food chains as distinctly modern, but not always foreign. In China, McDonald's restaurants were 50 percent Chinese owned, nearly all were Chinese managed, and 95 percent of the food sold was sourced from China. Surveys revealed that a majority of the young customers even believed that Ronald McDonald was Chinese and lived in Beijing. Instead of changing China's family-oriented food culture, McDonald's made money by catering to it. Entire families were welcomed for parties and celebrations, with paper and pen provided for young children to write and draw. Teahouses and art galleries were common features as well. Customers were initially attracted to fast food restaurants in China because they had clean toilets, a benefit that competing local restaurants were soon pressured to provide as well.

The chains that do best are those that follow local dietary preferences. KFC outsells McDonald's in China because chicken is more of a staple in the traditional Chinese diet than beef. Subway offers kosher food in Israel; nearly all of their restaurants in Muslim countries are *halal*; and vegetarian beef-free and pork-free meals are offered in India. McDonald's has also enjoyed rapid growth in India, with 300 restaurants by 2018. In Hindu India, where cows are revered, Big Macs have been replaced on the menu by giant Veg Maharaja Macs, made with double corn-and-cheese patties.

In countries such as China and India, it is the rise of an urban middle class that has done the most to alter traditional eating practices. Multinational supermarkets and fast food chains expand to make money as soon as this underlying shift begins, speeding the trend along and shaping it in a Western direction, but urbanization and income growth would have changed eating patterns in these countries even without supermarkets or Western fast food.

12

ORGANIC AND LOCAL FOOD

What is organic food?

The label "organic" refers to a restricted method of food production. Organic food is produced without any human-made (i.e., synthetic) fertilizers, pesticides, or preservatives. In organic systems, farmers use a variety of methods that do not require synthetic substances. For example, soil fertility is maintained by planting legumes that fix nitrogen naturally, or by using animal-derived nutrients such as composted manure. Insects are controlled using biological methods (relying on birds or spiders that eat insect pests), or by using naturally occurring pesticides such as Bt (a soil bacterium) or pyrethrins (produced by chrysanthemums) or sabadilla (derived from the ground seeds of lilies). Weeds are controlled not with synthetic herbicides but with mechanical cultivation or mulching. In place of synthetic preservatives, organic foods are traditionally cured with salt.

These methods are not new. Prior to the development of synthetic nitrogen fertilizers in the early 20th century, all food production worldwide was de facto organic. Only in the 20th century did organic methods come to be classified as distinct from emerging modern methods and then given a distinct label (the original label was "biodynamic"). Organically grown foods are not to be confused with foods sold as "natural," which are minimally processed foods that do not contain manufactured ingredients such as refined sugar, food colorings, or flavorings. Foods can be natural but not organic, just as some highly processed manufactured foods can be organic but not natural.

What is the history of organic food?

The organic food movement began in Europe early in the 20th century, originally as a philosophical rejection of synthetic nitrogen fertilizer. In 1909, two German chemists, Fritz Haber and Carl Bosch, had discovered a method to capture atmospheric nitrogen for agricultural use by combining it with hydrogen under high temperature and pressure, resulting in ammonia. Believers in "vitalist" theories of philosophy, which assert that living things such as plants can only be properly nourished by the products of other living things (e.g., other plants or animal manure), rejected this method of capturing nitrogen. The strongest rejection came in Austria, where the philosopher Rudolf Steiner championed what he called biodynamic ("life force") farming, which meant growing crops with composted animal manure plus other preparations such as chamomile blossom and oak bark. Steiner's approach was favored by conservatives at the time; it was promoted in Germany under the Third Reich by Rudolf Hess and Heinrich Himmler, who had come to doubt the sustainability of using artificial fertilizer and advocated instead "agriculture in accordance with the laws of life."

Skepticism toward synthetic nitrogen fertilizer also emerged in England early in the 20th century, where Albert Howard and Lady Eve Balfour took the lead in arguing against what they considered "artificial manures." To the present day, organic farming has strong support within the English upper class, most notably from King Charles, who in 1986 converted his own Duchy Home Farm to a completely organic system. The name "organic farming" first appeared in a 1940 book written by the English aristocrat Walter James, a follower of Steiner, and it was then introduced in the United States in 1942, when the American J. I. Rodale, who had taken inspiration from Sir Albert Howard's writings, began publishing a magazine he titled *Organic Gardening and Farming*. Rodale was also a promoter of alternative health care methods, and in the 1950s he founded *Prevention* magazine.

Organic backyard gardening has always been popular, but organic commercial farming was at first hard to promote because organic production costs were high, especially in terms of human labor, and the demand for organic products was still low. For years, organic products were sold only in specialty markets or health stores. The organic option gained a slightly stronger following after Rachel Carson's compelling critique of synthetic pesticide use in her 1962 book, *Silent Spring*, but it was a subsequent rise of consumer concerns about pesticide residues on food, in the late 1980s, that brought the movement to commercial significance. A movement that began as a philosophical rejection of synthetic fertilizer was finally energized by food safety fears linked to synthetic pesticides.

Organic advocacy from both growers and consumers eventually led Congress, in 1990, to mandate the creation of a clear national standard for certifying and labeling organically grown products. The emergence of this credible certification and labeling standard triggered a rapid expansion of both organic production and sales. Foods that were certified organic could command a higher price in the marketplace, giving growers a commercial incentive to convert to organic production systems.

How is organic food regulated in the United States?

Organic foods are regulated under a National Organic Program (NOP) created in 2002 by the US Department of Agriculture (USDA). Under this program, foods can be labeled "organic" only if grown and handled by certified organic producers and processors. The certification is performed not by the USDA directly but by third-party government-accredited certifiers who charge a fee. Depending on the size of the farm, certification can cost from a few hundred to several thousand dollars in the first year; annual inspections represent an added cost, but USDA reimburses up to 75 percent of the certification costs for eligible operations.

Certification is based on a requirement that only "nonsynthetic" substances be used in food production and handling. Synthetic fertilizers and pesticides are generally prohibited, along with the use of sewage sludge for fertilizer, the use of irradiation to kill food pathogens, and the planting of genetically engineered seeds. The USDA's original proposal would have allowed the use of sewage sludge, irradiation, and genetically engineered seeds, but outraged advocates for organic food sent 275,000 letters of complaint, so the government agreed in the end to exclude all three. Farms must be free of all prohibited substances and practices for at least three years to qualify for certification. In animal production, any animals used for meat, milk, or eggs must be fed 100 percent organic feed, have access to the outdoors, and may not be given hormones or antibiotics. Certified handlers of food must use only organic ingredients and must prevent organic and nonorganic products from coming into contact with each other. The products marketed by certified growers and handlers are then entitled to carry a prominent logo that says "USDA Organic."

Once this system began operating in 2002, consumer confidence in the integrity of organic producers and retailers increased, and commercial sales began growing rapidly at annual rates originally above 15 percent, slowing to 7 percent (still a high rate of growth) by 2010. The organic sector nonetheless remains small in the United States. In 2017, only 1.8 percent of farm commodities produced in the United States were organic, and in 2018 products certified organic made up just 5.7 percent of all the food sold in retail channels. The organic share of the total American diet is actually smaller than this, since half of all food spending in the United States now takes place in restaurants, and organic menu items are still a rarity. Organically certified foods are grown on only one-half of 1 percent of harvested cropland in the United States.

Is most organic food grown on small farms?

Many individual farms in America's organic sector are still small and highly diversified, but most organic production now comes from large industrial-scale farms. When the new National Organic Program came into full effect in 2002, food stores specializing in organic products such as Whole Foods and Wild Oats expanded their operations. Like all supermarkets, these retailers sought out suppliers who could deliver a steady volume of high-quality products, uniformly packaged and on time, and at a consistent grade. Small, diverse organic farms could not meet these requirements, so highly specialized industrial-scale farms expanded to take over. Earthbound Farm in California started out with just 2.5 acres of organic raspberries in 1984, but now it manages 50,000 acres and has taken over 55 percent of the national market for organic packaged salad greens. In 2007, a *Time* magazine cover story explained that Big Organic had taken over the sector by adopting "the same industrial-size farming and long-distance-shipping methods as conventional agribusiness." By 2011, three-quarters of all production came from large farms with annual sales of more than $1 million.

Some organic egg and dairy operations have now grown so large that traditional supporters are driven to object. At one organic egg farm in Saranac, Michigan, each rectangular building holds about 180,000 birds, with three hens for each square foot of floor space. The "outdoor" area required for organic certification is only a roofed-over screened porch. Katherine Paul of the Organic Consumers Association complained in 2017 that this was "not at all what consumers expect of an organic farm."

The Cornucopia Institute, which defends the original small-farm organic vision, complains about "factory milk" produced on organic dairy farms that house thousands of un-pastured cows. Cornucopia has also tried to block organic certification for hydroponic tomatoes that are grown without any soil at all. Large numbers of small organic farms still sell their products through local farmers' markets, but this quickly became just a small part of total organic sales. By 2014, only 8 percent of organic sales in the United States were made directly to consumers at farmers' markets or through community-supported agriculture (CSA) farms. Over 80 percent of all organic sales in the United States were being made under brands owned by corporate conglomerates like ConAgra, H.J. Heinz, or Kellogg. The biggest retailers of organic foods are now Walmart, Costco, and Kroger. Despite this commercial expansion, organically grown foods have remained considerably more expensive than their conventional counterparts. In 2018 the Food Marketing Institute reported that the average retail price (by volume) for organic produce was 54 percent higher than for conventional produce. One USDA study showed that organic salad mix cost 60 percent more than conventional, organic milk 72 percent more, and organic eggs 82 percent more.

Is organic food more nutritious and safe?

Consumers who pay more to purchase organic foods do so for multiple reasons. With organic fruits and vegetables, the motivation is often to gain a nutritional advantage, or to avoid pesticide residues on food, or to increase farmworker safety and protect the environment. Purchasers of organic meats and other livestock products often want to avoid microbial contamination, excessive antibiotic use, and the confinement of animals that typifies conventional livestock operations.

Strictly on nutritional grounds, health professionals from outside the organic community have found little or no advantage from organic foods. Claims of superior nutrient content are nonetheless made by the Organic Center, an institution founded in 2002 to demonstrate the benefits of organic products. For example in 2008, the Organic Center published a review "confirming" the nutrient superiority of plant-based organic foods, showing that they contained more vitamin C and vitamin E and a higher concentration of polyphenols, such as flavonoids. This review was rebutted, however, by conventional nutritionists who explained that the Organic Center had used statistical results either not peer-reviewed or not significant in terms of human health. Organic milk from cows raised on grass may indeed contain 50 percent more beta-carotene, but there is so little beta-carotene in conventional milk that the resulting gain is only an extra 112 micrograms of beta-carotene per quart of milk, or less than 1 percent the quantity of beta-carotene found in a single medium-size baked sweet potato.

European health professionals have also rejected the nutritional benefit claims. Claire Williamson from the British Nutrition Foundation states, "From a nutritional perspective, there is currently not enough evidence to recommend organic foods over conventionally produced foods." In 2009, the *American Journal of Clinical Nutrition* published a study, commissioned by the British Food Standards Agency, of 162 scientific papers produced in the past 50 years on the health and diet benefits of organically grown foods and found no evidence of a benefit. The director of the study concluded, "Our review indicates that there is currently no evidence to support the selection of organically over conventionally-produced on the basis of nutritional superiority." In 2012, a review of data from 237 studies conducted through the Center for Health Policy at Stanford University, published in the *Annals of Internal Medicine*, concluded that there were no convincing differences between organic and conventional foods in nutrient content or health benefits.

The claim that organic food is safer due to lower pesticide residues is also suspect in the eyes of most health professionals. The Mayo Clinic has said, "Some people buy organic food to limit their exposure to [pesticide] residues. Most experts agree, however, that the amount of pesticides found on fruits and vegetables poses a very small health risk." Residues on food can be a significant problem in developing countries, where the spraying of pesticides is poorly regulated and where fruits and vegetables are often sold unwashed, straight from the field. Yet in advanced industrial countries such as the United States, foods sold through commercial channels have residue levels that present only the smallest risk to health. In 2003, the Food and Drug Administration (FDA) analyzed several thousand samples of domestic and imported foods in the US market-place and found that only 0.4 percent of the domestic samples and only 0.5 percent of the imported samples had detectable chemical residues that exceeded the regulatory tolerance levels set by the UN through the Food and Agriculture Organization (FAO) and the World Health Organization (WHO).

These tolerance levels intentionally err on the side of caution. The UN establishes acceptable daily intake (ADI) levels for each separate pesticide, set conservatively at 1/100th of an exposure that still does not cause toxicity in laboratory animals. Actual exposure levels on marketed foods, in turn, are almost always far below the ADI level. When the FDA surveyed the highest exposures to 38 chemicals in the diets of various population subgroups in the United States, it found that for 4 of these 38 chemicals, the highest exposures were still less than 5 percent of the ADI level. For the other 34 chemicals, exposures were even lower, less than 1 percent of the ADI level. Carl K. Winter and Sarah F. Davis, food scientists at the University of California–Davis and the Institute of Food Technologies, conclude from these data, "[T]he marginal benefits of reducing human exposure to pesticides in the diet through increased consumption of organic produce appear to be insignificant."

Some advocacy organizations nonetheless continue to promote residue fears. The Environmental Working Group (EWG) still produces an annual "Dirty Dozen" report, listing the fruits and vegetables with the highest pesticide residue levels. Strawberries and spinach were at the top of the list in 2018. Of course, in any test of multiple products some will always be "dirtier" than others even when all are essentially clean. One paper published in 2011 looked at average pesticide exposures on that year's EWG "Dirty Dozen" products, and found all were well below a dose EPA might worry about, with the vast majority below 0.01 percent of this EPA reference dose.

It is true that conventional foods are sometimes not safe to consume, but organically grown foods can also carry risks. In 2006, bagged fresh spinach from a California farm in its final year of converting to organic certification was the source of *E. coli* infections in the United States that killed at least three and sickened hundreds. In 2009, there were nine documented fatal episodes of salmonella poisoning from peanut butter and ground peanut products traced to peanut plants in Texas and Georgia, both of which had organic certification. In 2011, 53 people died from eating bean sprouts that were organically grown in Germany yet were contaminated with *E. coli* bacteria.

Is organic farming better for the environment?

Organic farming systems are in some ways better for protecting the natural environment but in other ways they may be worse. As a general rule, organic systems are less likely to generate damaging chemical runoff and groundwater pollution, yet they will require the clearing of more land for every bushel of production, which makes them a threat—if scaled up—to forests, fragile lands, and wildlife habitat.

In the United States, according to USDA surveys of actual farms, yields per acre for organic row crops and vegetables are only 40–80 percent as high as the conventional average. This means that organic farms must plant much more land to secure each bushel of production. The same is true in Europe, where organically grown cereal crops have yields only 60–70 percent as high as those conventionally grown. In the UK, organic winter wheat yields are only 4 tons per hectare compared to 8 tons per hectare for conventional farms. The EU will confront this problem if it tries to make good on its 2021 "Farm to Fork" plan to increase organic acreage from 8 percent up to "at least" 25 percent by 2030.

Europe is embracing this strategy in part to fight climate change, but life-cycle assessments that take into account emissions from the livestock needed to produce the organic manure, plus the larger area of farmed land needed per ton of production, reveal that organic systems are not more climate friendly. Land use change is already the biggest source of greenhouse gas emissions from agriculture, and a switch from conventional methods to organic, which requires more land, makes this problem worse. One German study found that the expansion of cropland in Europe required by a shift to organic would eliminate 1.5 million hectares of European forest plus an additional 5 million hectares beyond Europe when other countries expanded cropland and production to meet Europe's enlarged food import needs.

Organic food is often promoted as friendly to the environment because there is no synthetic fertilizer or pesticide use. This is correct, yet the assertion must be qualified because organic farmers who overapply or mismanage animal waste can also pollute groundwater and surface water. In addition, when organic farmers control weeds by spreading a "mulch" carpet of black plastic that does not biodegrade, they create a new waste stream that must be loaded into dumpsters and taken to a landfill.

The uncertain environmental benefit from organic farming was confirmed in a 2012 report by scientists at Oxford University, published in the *Journal of Environmental Management*. Based on findings from 71 peer-reviewed studies, this report concluded that organic systems might be better for the environment per unit of land, but conventional systems were often better per unit of food production. By implication, as production requirements increase the environmental cost of employing organic methods will increase as well.

The best farming systems for the environment are those that integrate conventional and organic methods. For example, soil health is often best protected when prudent quantities of synthetic chemical fertilizers are used in combination with cover crops, crop rotations, and manure. Yet this is a best practice blocked by the rigid organic standard, because the use of any synthetic nitrogen at all is strictly prohibited. Pest control is best accomplished through integrated pest management methods that begin with natural biological controls but allow careful applications of chemical insecticides as a last resort, yet even the smallest use of synthetic chemicals is blocked under the organic standard. The strict prohibition against synthetic herbicide use in organic farming also holds back the use of no-till practices, which are a superior method for avoiding soil erosion, burning less diesel fuel, sequestering carbon, and reducing greenhouse gas emissions. The organic standard also makes it impossible to plant genetically engineered crops such as Bt corn and Bt cotton, which help conventional farmers reduce insecticide use. Environmental protection was not the original motive for advocating organic methods a century ago, so these environmental limitations embedded in the organic standard today should not be surprising.

Could today's world be fed with organically grown food?

Assuming current levels of consumption, it is no longer possible to provide the world with its current diet using only organic farming systems that prohibit the use of synthetic nitrogen fertilizer. In the past century, the population of the earth has increased from 1.6 billion to 8 billion, and these much larger numbers are being fed thanks largely to the higher crop yields made possible by synthetic nitrogen. Since the 1930s, for example, wheat yields in conventional farming using nitrogen fertilizer have doubled. Vaclav Smil, an agronomist from the University of Manitoba, calculates that synthetic fertilizers currently supply about 40 percent of all the nitrogen used by crops around the world. To replace this synthetic nitrogen with organic nitrogen would require the manure production of approximately 7–8 billion additional cattle, roughly a fivefold increase from current numbers, creating an unacceptable environmental burden.

Advocates for organic farming, such as the International Federation of Organic Agricultural Movements, do not frame the problem this way. They assert that organic practices can increase yields, pointing to farming projects they have carried out in some of the world's hungriest regions, such as Africa. For documentation they refer to a 2006 meta-study in the journal *Renewable Agriculture and Food Systems* and to a 2008 UN report titled *Organic Agriculture and Food Security in Africa*. Yet most of the yield claims made in these studies are based on project-level comparisons between improved organic systems and traditional systems with no soil improvements at all, rather than comparisons between organic and conventionally fertilized "green revolution" systems.

Many of Africa's smallholder farmers today are actually de facto organic, because they use no synthetic fertilizers or pesticides, but this has not made them more productive. Certified organic farming has expanded in Africa in recent years, but mostly to grow crops for export to supermarkets in Europe, rather than to provide food for local consumption.

What is the local food movement?

When organic farming in the United States began taking on a large-scale industrial appearance, disillusioned advocates began to promote local food, since it would more often be purchased directly from smaller growers at farmers' markets, community gardens, co-ops, or through CSA subscriptions.

The social movement to promote this kind of locally grown food was first consolidated in the United States in 2005, when Jessica Prentice, the founder of a community-supported kitchen in Berkeley, California, coined the term "locavore" to describe those who opt to get their food, when possible, from within a 100-mile radius (the "100-mile diet"). It became clear that significant numbers of consumers were willing to pay more for locally grown food, so farmers' markets and local CSAs began to proliferate, retail stores and restaurants began to label locally sourced products as such, and schools and restaurants began developing "farm to school" and "farm to table" relationships with local growers. Suburban communities lifted some of their restrictions on backyard livestock production, and municipal authorities began promoting various kinds of "urban agriculture" to allow local purchase.

The local food movement brought a significant expansion in direct farmer-to-customer sales. Between 2005 and 2016, according to the USDA, the number of farmers' markets in operation in America increased from 4,000 up to more than 20,000. Yet the total share of America's marketed food that can be called "local" remained small. According to the 2017 Census of Agriculture, the market value of all farm sales made directly to consumers at farmers' markets and CSAs, or farm to school and farm to table, plus sales through food hubs for local or regionally branded products, made up only 3 percent of national farm sales. If we take into consideration the imported foods in our diet that are grown by farmers abroad, this locally grown share becomes even smaller.

There is no single agreed-upon definition of "local" food. The USDA describes a food product as local or regional if it either comes from in-state, or from within a 400-mile radius, which is a distance four times as great as the movement's leaders would prefer. When labeling its products "locally grown," Walmart uses the in-state definition. Whole Foods uses a time-in-transit standard (seven or fewer hours of travel by car or truck) but the company allows individual stores to use tighter rules if they wish.

What explains the attraction of local food to consumers?

Surveys reveal that consumers are willing to pay more for locally grown food (roughly 12 percent more for local tomatoes) because they believe local means fresher, because they want to support their local economy, because they want to know where their food did or did not come from, and also because they want to support small farms as opposed to industrial-scale farms. Some consumers also believe local food will be more nutritious and safer to eat than supermarket food, and will emit less greenhouse gas because it will travel fewer miles.

The nutrition advantage can be real, because locally grown food sold at a farmers' market is more likely to have been picked recently, closer to optimal ripeness. As a disadvantage, most local food is only available in season, so in colder regions buying locally will be an excellent supplement to good nutrition during warm months, but with limitations in winter. Regarding safety, locally grown food is ordinarily just as safe as supermarket food, but seldom any safer. Spoilage of meat is as much of a problem when buying from small local producers as when buying from supermarkets. Produce from farmers' markets is sometimes less thoroughly washed, and the marketing surfaces may be less thoroughly sanitized. Local raw-milk cheese may be just as likely to carry listeria. Small local producers often lack the costly equipment used by larger operations to protect against microbial contamination. In 2010, local growers who engaged in direct sales demanded from Congress—and were given—an exemption from some of the new food safety requirements that others would have to observe.

Direct food sales from farmers to local consumers can certainly bring important social benefits. Some consumers purchase food from farmers' markets or CSAs simply to add a satisfying social dimension to their weekly food routine. Sociologists calculate that shoppers will have on average 10 times as many conversations at a farmers' market compared to a supermarket. Journalist Michael Pollan, a leading voice in the local food movement, has observed that when people shop at a farmers' market they become less like consumers and more like neighbors. "In many cities and towns," he wrote in

2010, "farmers' markets have taken on (and not for the first time) the function of a lively new public square."

Political support for the local food movement has grown strong enough in the United States to inspire a number of supporting federal programs, including a Community Food Project Grants Program for CSAs, a voucher program for low-income seniors to shop at farmers' markets, a Commodity Facilities Program to support construction of farmers' markets, and in 2009 a USDA initiative from the Obama administration named "Know Your Farmer, Know Your Food" that funneled $1 billion into infrastructure projects for local food and farm-to-school grants. Advocates for local food in 2009 persuaded First Lady Michelle Obama to visit a farmers' market near the White House, and then plant an organic vegetable garden on the White House lawn. In 2022, the Biden administration announced a $400 million program to create "regional food business centers" plus an initial $75 million to support urban agriculture. Democratic administrations tend to provide greater support for local food systems, because these systems are more likely to be led by Democrats, while Republicans tend to favor the long-distance, industrial food systems that generally support them.

Is urban agriculture a promising alternative?

One innovative branch of the local food movement is enthusiasm for growing food in cities, either in community gardens on vacant lots, on rooftops, or on vertical structures inside buildings. The community gardens have a proven social value, even when they produce very little food, so they often enjoy strong financial support through city budgets and from philanthropic foundations. Rooftop farms and vertical indoor farms are more likely to pursue a commercial purpose such as growing leafy greens for local restaurants.

Urban community gardens can spring up quickly in cities where lots have become vacant due to industrial decline. In Detroit, space has been found for 1,300 neighborhood gardens growing 400,000 pounds of produce. RecoveryPark Farms has turned a 22-block area into a complex of hoop houses that grow leafy greens, herbs, and exotic vegetables for restaurants. This project, which serves people recovering from substance abuse, survives thanks to rent-free land provided by the city. In Camden, New Jersey, community gardens produce enough to feed about 500 people a day during the growing season. This isn't very many in a city of 80,000 people, but the gardens don't just provide food; they build social cooperation, discipline, and community leadership.

Rooftop and indoor farms strive for success in the commercial marketplace. The Brooklyn Grange in New York is a for-profit rooftop farm that grows vegetables for sale through its own CSA, and also at local farmstands and to local restaurants. It supplements this income by renting its garden spaces (which have spectacular views of the Manhattan skyline) for private dinners and weddings. America's largest indoor vertical farm is AeroFarms, located in a former steel mill in Newark, New Jersey. Several indoor farms have run into financial trouble and had to close, including FarmedHere in Chicago, and a downtown farm in Vancouver.

Most of urban agriculture remains sub-commercial. A 2013 survey found that one-third of urban farms were not-for-profit, 20 percent were growing their products for donation, and 60 percent remained in operation thanks to fundraising, grants, or off-farm work. Commercial urban farms in New York City primarily produce leafy greens sold at prices only upscale consumers can afford, while providing only entry-level jobs paying less than a living wage. Costs are high because urban real estate is expensive, and energy costs for indoor LEDs are more expensive than sunlight.

Are localized food systems more resilient to shocks?

When the COVID-19 pandemic struck early in 2020, food systems around the world were placed under acute stress. Supply chain disruptions brought on by lockdowns and social distancing led to the temporary closing of many large meat processing plants, which gave livestock producers nowhere to sell their market-ready animals. This experience led advocates for local food to allege that a more localized food system would be more resilient to shocks of this kind. This in turn helped trigger a USDA initiative in 2022 to "shore up the food supply chain" in part by encouraging a more decentralized food system infrastructure, including $375 million to support smaller, independent meat and poultry processing plants.

In fact, America's long-distance (non-local) food system performed remarkably well during the COVID-19 stress test. The nation's food imports from abroad actually continued to increase during the pandemic, and the meat processing disruptions were modest overall and temporary. Pork processing in the second quarter of 2020 did fall 4 percent below the second quarter level of 2019, but then quickly recovered and for 2020 overall it was higher than in 2019, a production increase that continued in 2021. The biggest disruptions came, in the end, from the closure of schools and restaurants due to lockdown mandates, plus hoarding behavior by nervous supermarket shoppers, but it isn't clear how a more localized food system could have overcome either of these difficulties.

In the end, the best evidence that America's non-local food system showed resilience during the crisis came from USDA survey data on household food security. These data showed that food insecurity did not increase in 2020 compared to 2019, and the next year's data for 2021 showed the same thing.

The dominant food system trend continues to be globalization, not localization. US agricultural exports have grown steadily over the past quarter century—reaching $177 billion in 2021, up from $66.5 billion in 1996. On average between 2010 and 2020, more than 20 percent of America's agricultural products, both manufactured and non-manufactured, were exported. America's agricultural imports have grown even faster. Between 1996 and 2021, total agricultural imports more than quadrupled in value, reaching $171 billion in 2021.

On average, the United States imports 43 percent of its fruit and nuts and 34 percent of its vegetable consumption, with the overall imported share of food and beverage consumption, by value, growing from 13.1 percent in 2010 to 18.3 percent in 2020. Market forces such as falling shipping rates, and new technologies such as refrigerated shipping containers, have driven much of this growth in trade, but an equally large factor has been consumer demand for a constantly wider variety of food choices, particularly off-season during the cold winter months.

Would shifting to local food help slow climate change?

Claims that local food production cuts greenhouse gas emissions by reducing the burning of transportation fuel are usually not well founded. Transport is the source of only 11 percent of greenhouse gas emissions within the food sector, so reducing the distance that food travels after it leaves the farm is far less important than reducing wasteful energy use on the farm, and food coming from a distance can actually be better for the climate if produced with less fossil energy. For example, field-grown tomatoes shipped from Mexico in the winter months will have a smaller carbon footprint, per tomato, than local winter tomatoes grown in a heated greenhouse. In the UK, lamb meat that travels 11,000 miles from New Zealand generates only one-quarter the carbon emissions per pound compared to British lamb, because farmers in the UK raise their animals on feed (which must be produced using fossil fuels) rather than on clover pastureland.

When food does travel, what matters most is not the distance traveled but the travel mode (surface versus air), and most of all the load size. Bulk loads of food can travel halfway around the world by ocean freight with a smaller carbon footprint, per pound delivered, than foods traveling just a short distance but in much smaller loads. For example, compared to small-load pickup trucks, large-load 18-wheelers can move food 100 times as far while burning only one-third as much gas per pound of food delivered. Local growers who move food around in small loads by pickup are burning far more fossil fuel, per tomato delivered, than large growers from out of state who move food around in bulk.

What is the difference between local food and slow food?

The slow food movement (whose logo is a snail) originated in Italy in 1986, initially as a backlash against the introduction of fast foods into Europe. Slow food advocates work to preserve local cuisines and gastronomic traditions, including heirloom varieties of local grains and breeds of livestock. They view this as one way to fight back against the loss of culture and the more frenzied lifestyle introduced by fast foods, supermarkets, and global agribusiness. Slow food is now an important international social movement, with roughly 100,000 members organized into more than 1,500 local chapters (called *convivia*) in 160 different countries. Each *convivium* promotes local farmers, local food artisans, and local Taste Workshops.

Compared to Italians, most Americans are less concerned with gastronomic traditions, but in 2008, more than 60,000 people attended a slow food gathering in San Francisco, savoring local cuisines at taste pavilions and celebrating the planting of an urban garden in front of City Hall. In 2010, thousands of local slow food supporters participated in nationwide "Dig Ins," by first gardening together and then eating together. In 2021, Slow Food USA supported donations of 250 rare seed kits to school gardens.

What explains the loyalty of some groups to organic, local, or slow food?

Groups in society have always sought solidarity through the foods they eat, or the foods they agree not to eat. Within most religious traditions, patterns of food consumption are carefully regulated. Judaism has strict rules, called *kashrut*, to specify what may and may not be eaten. In Islam, foods are divided into *haram* (forbidden) and *halal* (permitted). Hindus who embrace the concept of *ahimsa* do not eat meat to avoid doing violence to animals. In Roman Catholicism, fasting is required and meat consumption is discouraged at certain times in the religious calendar.

In today's less religious world, we should not be surprised to see the emergence of informal food rules within more secular settings, to pursue and express social solidarity around shared practices and values. The new rules that emerge (organic, local, or slow) may be attractive or practical only for relatively small subcategories of citizens, or perhaps only for a small part of the diet of those citizens, but the exclusivity and the extra effort required by the rule can be part of its attraction. The goal is to express through the diets we adopt a solidarity with others who share our identity, our values, or our particular life circumstances. The scientific foundation for these modern food rules may sometimes be weak, but the social value can nonetheless be strong.

13

FOOD SAFETY AND GENETICALLY ENGINEERED FOODS

How safe is America's food supply?

In rich countries, the food choices available in supermarkets and restaurants are almost always free from dangerous levels of toxic or microbial contamination. Even when they are not healthful or nutritious, they deserve to be called "safe." In the United States, food safety risks are low—in fact, lower than ever—yet as societies become more affluent, even a small risk can be seen as unacceptable. Food safety lapses continue to be big stories in the popular media, and both food companies and food retailers know they will pay a heavy price if a lapse can be traced back to them.

Food can be a source of more than 200 known diseases, because it exposes us to viruses, bacteria, parasites, toxins, metals, and prions (as in the case of mad cow disease). Food illness symptoms can range from mild gastroenteritis to life-threatening neurologic, hepatic, and renal syndromes. According to the Centers for Disease Control and Prevention (CDC), food-borne diseases cause 1 in 6 Americans to be sick each year, 128,000 to be hospitalized, and approximately 3,000 to die. Three pathogens, salmonella, listeria, and toxoplasma, are responsible for approximately 30 percent of the deaths. Children under the age of four are sickened by food more than any other age group, but adults over the age of 50 suffer more hospitalizations and deaths.

The changing frequency of food-borne illness in any large population is difficult to monitor and measure. Mild cases often go unreported, so official frequency counts will be heavily dependent on the intensity of surveillance. Nationally since 1996, the CDC has attempted to track food-borne sickness through regular surveys of more than 650 clinical laboratories around the country that serve about 46 million people in 10 different states. At the state level, surveillance is less systematic, leading to counts that are hard to compare. Food-borne illness can even be overreported, because many pathogens transmitted by food may also be spread through water or from person to person without anything being ingested at all. Specific pathogens may never be identified, creating a further possibility that an illness was unrelated to food.

America's food supply is far safer today than it was in the past, before the era of refrigeration and sanitary packaging. Surveys by the CDC show decades of steadily increasing safety up to the present day for some common infections. For example, infections caused by E. coli O157 declined by 44 percent between 1996 and 2010, while infections from listeria declined 38 percent and campylobacter by 27 percent. Infections from salmonella, however, were no longer declining and had even increased by 3 percent between 1996 and 2010. The CDC attributes the overall downward trend in food-borne infections to enhanced knowledge about how to prevent contaminations, cleaner slaughter methods, increased awareness in food service establishments and private homes of the risks of undercooked ground beef, and the regulatory prohibition, since 1994, of any contamination of ground beef with E. coli O157.

The COVID-19 emergency brought CDC numbers on food-borne illness down even more. During 2020, observed incidences of infections decreased by an additional 26 percent compared to 2017–2019. The CDC attributed this to changes in daily life due to lockdowns plus hygiene behaviors such as handwashing that reduced exposure to food-borne pathogens, plus some decreased detection of infections due to fewer visits to the doctor.

The vast majority of hospitalizations and fatalities from food contamination today come not from large outbreaks linked to dangerous batches of products in supermarkets but instead from a steady background level of illness caused by careless handling and improper preparation inside the home. Unwashed hands, unwashed cutting boards, poorly refrigerated foods, or insufficiently cooked meats are the most frequent cause. Wider illness outbreaks still take place, but the fatalities are usually quite limited. For example, illness from bagged spinach in 2006 led to a nationwide scare and the virtual suspension of all fresh and bagged spinach sales in America, but there were only three known deaths. In 2011, listeria on melons from Colorado caused the single worst food-borne disease outbreak since 1985, but with only 33 known deaths. Consumers fear contamination in meats, but in the United States twice as many people are likely to get sick from contaminated produce versus contaminated meat.

Assuming the CDC number of 3,000 annual deaths from food-borne illness is accurate, this is far fewer than the 300,000 annual deaths caused by diseases linked to obesity. Eating *too much* food is now a significantly greater health risk in America than eating unsafe food. Yet any illness from foods contaminated at purchase will cause public outrage, because this is an involuntary exposure to risk, unlike risks from overeating, or smoking. Because purchasing food at supermarkets is a common experience for us all, anxieties spread quickly when a danger in the market is confirmed or even rumored. The unusually wide audience for these fears explains why the popular media give food contamination outbreaks such sensational coverage. Under the spotlight of media attention, government officials and politicians are always obliged to express intense concern, whatever the actual magnitude of the problem.

How do foods become contaminated?

Food is vulnerable to contamination at nearly every stage along the production and delivery chain, all the way from farm to fork. Microbial contamination of fresh produce is possible at the farm level (a problem with California lettuce and Guatemalan raspberries in the 1990s). In meat slaughter, inadequate knife sterilization and improper evisceration or hide removal can lead to contamination. Pathogens can also be introduced by unsanitary conveyor belts or unclean processing and packaging equipment. Farther down the chain in wholesale and retail outlets, inadequate refrigeration can be a problem. In restaurants, cooks who do not wash their hands introduce risks.

Private food companies have learned to minimize contamination through the use of what are called Hazard Analysis and Critical Control Point (HACCP) systems. These systems, first innovated by the Pillsbury Company in the 1960s, identify where hazards might enter the food production process and specify the stringent actions needed at each separate step to prevent this from occurring. In 1996, the US Department of Agriculture (USDA) issued its own rule for HACCP systems for meat and poultry, a requirement that was costly for industry, but effective, as suggested by the 44 percent reduction in *E. coli* O157 contamination seen since 1996. Protection against contamination took another step forward in 2022, when the FDA published a final rule governing "traceability protocols" that certain operators in the food supply chain will have to follow (small farms are exempted). These will be recordkeeping requirements to make it easier to trace and remove contaminated items. The new rule comes into effect in 2026.

Food adulteration is a related issue. Consumers will spurn foods if they are found to contain ingredients not indicated on the label, especially ingredients of lower quality, even if the food is perfectly safe to consume. Ground meats are often sold containing safe ingredients that would nonetheless surprise and even anger consumers, if they knew. In 2012, many American consumers were distressed to learn, from an ABC news broadcast, that a product extracted from slaughterhouse beef trimmings known as "pink slime" was being used in ground beef. There was no demonstrated safety risk, but some companies halted the sale of ground beef that used this filler, in an effort to reassure consumers. In 2013 in Europe, a discovery that some ground beef products contained more than 1 percent horse meat led to the withdrawal of millions of products from supermarkets in Ireland, the UK, France, Italy, Spain, Sweden, and Romania.

In poorly regulated food systems, food adulteration can be extremely dangerous. In 2008, manufacturers in China added melamine (a synthetic chemical often used in plastics that has a high nitrogen content) to infant formula to make it seem as though their products had enough protein. This led to kidney failure in babies, and news reports indicated the fraud caused over 300,000 illnesses, 50,000 hospitalizations, and at least 6 deaths.

Who regulates food contamination in the United States?

At the federal level, responsibility for food safety is divided between the Food and Drug Administration (FDA) inside the US Department of Health and Human Services, and the Food Safety and Inspection Service (FSIS) inside the USDA. The FSIS is responsible for meat and poultry, while the FDA is responsible for everything else. State public health agencies and city and county health departments also play a continuous monitoring role. Inadequate coordination among these various agencies has been a persistent concern, and in 1998, the Clinton administration created a Food Outbreak Response Coordinating Group inside the Department of Health and Human Services, designed to increase communication and coordination. The division of labor between the FSIS and the FDA has nonetheless remained problematic. For example, frozen pizzas are inspected by the FDA if they are cheese, and by the FSIS if they are pepperoni. The FSIS is responsible for chickens, but the FDA is responsible for eggs.

Within FDA, food safety sometimes gets less focused attention than drug safety. In 2022, critics called on the FDA commissioner to appoint a single individual, in a deputy commissioner position, to be in charge of all of the food programs of the agency. Others have suggested moving the food programs of the agency to the USDA.

Food industries in the United States are generally comfortable with strong FDA safety regulations. Following a highly publicized salmonella outbreak in eggs in 2010, which sickened people in all 50 states (though no one died), Congress passed a new food safety law (the Food Safety Modernization Act, the first major change since 1938), giving the FDA new responsibilities to inspect food processing plants and farms for prevention purposes, rather than just tracing contamination after it occurs. This new law had bipartisan support from Republicans as well as Democrats, and from food industries as well as from consumer protection advocates. Food industries liked the law because it offered help in avoiding broad product recalls. Following the 2006 *E. coli* spinach outbreak, which was traced to a single farm, total retail sales of bagged spinach dropped $202 million over the following 68-week period. After a 2009 salmonella contamination in peanut butter (traced to a single processing plant in Georgia), Kellogg had to recall peanut-containing products worth $70 million. Big food companies typically resist tougher rules when it comes to labeling for dietary health, but they welcome assistance from the FDA in preserving food safety, for their own self-protection.

In fact, something of a de facto partnership between consumer advocates and big food companies surfaced in 2012, when budget cutters in the House of Representatives threatened to deny the FDA the funds it would need to implement the new 2010 law. This threat was turned back through a joint lobbying effort by consumer protection advocates plus a range of big food trade associations, including the Grocery Institute, the Snack Food Association, and the Produce Marketing Association. In the end, the budget for the FDA's new food safety program was increased rather than cut, and in early 2013 the agency proposed a sweeping array of new rules covering all aspects of growing and harvesting produce, including threats from animal manure, worker hygiene, and water use. The compliance cost was estimated at $460 a year for US farmers and $1.2 billion a year for food processors.

Is food safety an issue in international trade?

Food safety often emerges as a concern in international trade, but the risks are sometimes exaggerated by national industries seeking protection from foreign competition. Imported foods from countries with a history of lax safety standards, such as China, are a genuine concern. The United States imports a considerable volume of food products from China every year, mostly seafood, juices, and pickled, dried, or canned vegetables. Prior to the enactment of a new food safety law in 2009, China had a notoriously bad food safety record, as illustrated by the 2008 infant formula scandal. In addition, Chinese peaches had been found preserved with sodium metabisulfite, rice was contaminated with cadmium, noodles were flavored with ink and paraffin, mushrooms were treated with fluorescent bleach, and cooking oil was recycled from street gutters.

Fortunately for importers of Chinese products, most of these poorly regulated foods were excluded from export channels. Chinese authorities work hard to control the safety of products that enter the world market by maintaining separate certification both for exporters and for the farms that supply them. A second line of defense for the United States is the FDA, which physically inspects only 2 percent of food imports into the United States but screens all imports electronically using an automated system that helps identify products posing the greatest risk. The FDA has offices in China—in Beijing, Shanghai, and Guangzhou—tasked with identifying potential food safety problems before shipments depart for the United States. Federal funding for surveillance of the nation's food supply increased after the 9/11 attacks, following enactment of a 2002 Bioterrorism Preparedness and Response Act, which deputized the Department of Homeland Security to assist in enforcing FDA standards, especially at ports of entry into the country.

When imported foods are found to be unsafe, the political reaction is often excessive. In 1989, when the FDA announced that it had found two grapes from Chile contaminated with cyanide, it banned imports of all Chilean fruits, costing Chilean exporters more than $400 million. In 2001, the USDA banned $278 million in annual imports of live hogs and uncooked animal products from Europe, to stem the spread of foot-and-mouth disease; the motives were clearly mixed, since US meat producers had been seeking such a ban for years to punish Europe for refusing to accept hormone-treated meat from the United States. In 2011 when an outbreak of E. coli in German sprouts killed 53 people, nearly all in Germany, the Germans initially tried to blame the outbreak on cucumbers from Spain. This damaged the reputation of Spanish exporters and cost them $200 million a week in lost sales. Russia then banned the import of all fresh vegetables from the entire EU.

Does the industrialization of agriculture make food less safe?

The industrialization of agriculture does not make food more dangerous overall, but it does present new kinds of safety risks. In the past, food contamination outbreaks were more frequent but usually localized and small-scale; today, outbreaks are far less frequent (per unit of food) yet much harder to contain in one local area when they do occur. Outbreaks spread quickly today to multiple states, attracting national media attention and creating an impression that our modern food system is less safe than a more compartmentalized or localized alternative.

For example, the worst food safety lapse in recent US history was a 2011 outbreak of listeria in cantaloupe, traced to a single packing shed in Colorado. It sickened 123 people in 26 states and actually killed 33. Yet the 33 fatalities from this largest industrial farming failure were just a tiny fraction of that year's 3,000 estimated fatalities from food-borne illness overall. Most fatalities from unsafe food still take place due to lapses inside private homes, and localized and traditional food systems can fail more often because they are less able to afford state-of-the-art technical options for food supply protection.

Is irradiated food safe?

One method for reducing or eliminating harmful bacteria, insects, and parasites in food is to irradiate the food with brief exposures to X-rays, gamma rays, or an electron beam. This technique has been known for the better part of a century, yet it remains rarely used in the United States. The FDA approved irradiation as safe and effective for use on poultry in 1992, and on meat in 1997, but it is rarely used because it makes the meat more costly and because the industry fears an adverse consumer response to the word "radiation." In the United States, irradiated foods must be labeled with a symbol, plus the words "treated with irradiation." In 2001, the CDC estimated that if half the nation's meat and poultry supply were irradiated, the result would be 900,000 fewer annual cases of food-borne illness and 350 fewer deaths. Advocates for irradiation observe that the technique has been judged safe by the government and might have killed the salmonella that reached grocery store shelves early in 2009 in peanut butter and peanut paste. Critics say that irradiation would only be used by private companies to hide the filthy condition of their plants.

What are genetically modified foods?

Nearly all foods come from plants and animals with genes that have been modified over time by human actions ranging from simple seed selections by farmers to scientific plant breeding. In current usage, however, the term "genetically modified" is reserved for plants or animals modified through genetic engineering, using the science of recombinant DNA (rDNA). This method, first practiced in 1973, modifies plants and animals not through controlled sexual reproduction but instead by moving individual genes physically from a source organism directly into the living DNA of a target organism. The value of this technique comes from its relative precision and its access to a wider pool of genetic resources. For example, genes carrying a specific trait to resist insect damage can be moved from a soil bacterium named Bt into a corn plant or into a cotton plant. The modified versions of these plants are known as Bt corn and Bt cotton. Alternatively, genes that direct a plant to produce beta-carotene (a precursor of vitamin A, which helps prevent blindness) can be moved from a daffodil plant into a rice plant, resulting in something called "Golden Rice."

The first engineered crop approved for commercial sale was a tomato with extended shelf life (the FlavrSavr tomato), approved by FDA and marketed by the Calgene Company in 1994. Then, in 1995, the Monsanto Company secured approval for sale in the United States of Roundup Ready soybean plants, engineered to resist the herbicide glyphosate (sold by Monsanto under the trade name Roundup), which simplified the problem of weed control. With one application of glyphosate, the weeds would die, but the soybean plants would not. By 1996, Monsanto's Bt corn and Bt cotton had also been approved for commercial use in the United States. The EU also approved a number of genetically engineered crops for both human consumption and planting in 1995–1996, including soybean, maize (corn), and canola; Japan approved soybean and tomato; Argentina approved soybean and maize; Australia approved cotton and canola; and, in 1995–1996, Mexico approved soybean, canola, potato, and tomato.

How are genetically engineered foods regulated?

Each national government has its own system for approving the planting and consumption of genetically engineered crops and foods. The United States, from the start, regulated genetically engineered crops and foods in much the same manner that it regulated conventional crops and foods, based on a 1987 National Academy of Sciences finding that there was no evidence of "unique hazards" from the modification of plants using rDNA methods versus other methods. All new crops in the United States, including genetically engineered crops, are subject to regulation for biosafety (safety to the biological environment, especially to other agricultural crops and animals) by the Animal and Plant Health Inspection Service (APHIS) of the USDA. If a crop has been engineered to produce a pesticide (such as Bt), the Environmental Protection Agency (EPA) must give its approval. The FDA is the agency that reviews new genetically engineered crops for food safety. The FDA will consider the genetically engineered varieties of familiar foods to be no less safe than the conventional varieties of those same foods, so long as the engineering process has not introduced a new or unfamiliar toxicant, nutrient, or allergenic protein. Technology developers consult with the FDA to share the results of their own safety testing (the consultation is voluntary, but all developers do it); then they can put the new product on the market.

Governments in Europe have a different approach to regulating genetically engineered crops and foods, known there as genetically modified organisms (GMOs). The European approach, which many other governments around the world have also followed, is to create separate laws and separate approval procedures for GMOs, and also to regulate this technology according to a far more demanding standard. Regulators in Europe can block the approval of a GMO without any evidence of an actual risk to human health or the environment, under what is known as the "precautionary principle." A new technology can be blocked on suspicion of a risk not yet tested for, or because of fear that a risk not found in the short run might still show up in the long run.

Despite this more precautionary approach, EU regulatory authorities did approve a number of GMO foods and crops in 1995–1996, as mentioned above. Fear of GMOs grew in Europe, however, following a 1996 "mad cow disease" scandal in the UK. This disease was scientifically unrelated to GMOs but it undercut citizen confidence in government food safety regulators. European regulators needed to restore their credibility with consumers, so they became more cautious toward all food technologies, especially GMOs. In 1998, yielding to demands from European activist groups such as Greenpeace and Friends of the Earth, they imposed an informal moratorium on any new approvals of GMOs. A number of European governments even began rejecting GMOs that had earlier been approved by EU authorities.

Finally, in 2004, the EU introduced a new set of regulations intended to reassure consumers through strict labeling plus the tracing of any approved GMO food through the marketplace. Henceforth, all GMO products with as much as 0.9 percent transgenic content would have to carry an identifying label, and operators in the food chain handling these approved GMOs would have to maintain audit trails, for at least five years, showing where each GM product came from and to whom it had been sold. Instead of reassuring consumers, these tight regulations reinforced popular suspicion that the technology must be dangerous in some way. Food companies in Europe responded by voluntarily taking GMO ingredients out of their products, in order to avoid stigmatizing labels.

How widespread are genetically engineered foods?

As of 2019, 29 countries around the world had approved at least some genetically engineered crops for planting, and 43 additional countries had approved imports of at least some for food, feed, or processing rather than planting. At total of

190.4 million acres were planted to such crops, up from 170 million acres in 2012. Still, this uptake has remained limited both by geography and by crop variety. In 2019, 84 percent of all these GMO crop acres were in just four Western Hemisphere countries: the United States, Brazil, Argentina, and Canada. In addition, 97.2 percent of total GMO acres were planted to just four crops: soybeans, maize, cotton, and canola. Soybeans and yellow maize are used primarily for oil, biofuel, or animal feed; cotton is an industrial crop; and canola is typically crushed for oil or meal, so none of these dominant GMO crops provided a staple food for direct human consumption. In response to consumer fears, staple foods such as rice, wheat, and potato have scarcely been grown anywhere in genetically engineered form.

Even in the United States, the leading GMO country, consumer anxieties at home and abroad have blocked the commercialization of most GMO food crops. It is estimated that roughly 70 percent of foods in the United States contain some ingredients from GMOs, but most of those ingredients are derivative products from soy or maize, such as oil, meal, sweeteners, or starch. As of 2022, no GMO wheat or rice was being grown commercially in the United States, and the only GMO fruits or vegetables grown commercially were papaya (in Hawaii), some summer squash, and some sweet corn. GMO potatoes were grown on 25,000 acres in the United States between 1999 and 2001, but then cultivation was voluntarily suspended when food service chains such as McDonald's and Burger King told suppliers they did not want to be accused by activists of serving GMO French fries. GMO tomatoes were also cultivated commercially in the United States between 1998 and 2002, but when consumer anxieties increased, they too were voluntarily withdrawn.

In most other countries, the absence of GMO crop production is a result of explicit regulatory blockage. As of 2022 in all of Sub-Saharan Africa, the only three countries where it was fully legal for farmers to plant any GMO crops were the Republic of South Africa, Burkina Faso (cotton only), and Nigeria (cotton and cowpea). In much of Sub-Saharan Africa, it is not yet legal even to do research on GMO crops. In Tanzania in 2018, a confined government research trial of drought-tolerant Bt maize was officially shut down after controversies arose, and the planting materials were ordered destroyed.

Both India and China have invested public resources in developing GMO crops, but so far Bt cotton is the only crop fully approved for cultivation in India, and the only GMO crop widely cultivated in China. Official biosafety committees in these countries approved two new GMO food crops in 2009 (eggplant in India and rice in China), but in India the approval was immediately blocked through the intervention of the environment minister, and in China senior political authorities decided not to approve GMO rice. By 2022 it seemed likely that China would soon approve GMO soybean and maize, to help meet growing livestock feed requirements.

Why do some people resist GMOs?

Opposition to genetically engineered foods and crops is framed by some as a defense of food safety or environmental safety, by others as a defense of the rights of traditional farming communities, and by still others as resistance against the profit-making companies that develop and patent the technology. Others object because they think that the technology has been inadequately regulated, or because GMO foods are not adequately labeled in the marketplace.

These concerns are frequently fueled by sensational claims and charges. For years critics asserted that GMOs produced sterile seeds, forcing farmers to buy seeds every year. Others believed that GMOs killed butterflies, or created superbugs and superweeds, or threatened biodiversity. Others believed that GMOs required an increased use of chemical sprays. Others believed rats that were fed GMOs had developed tumors. Still others believed that biotechnology companies—specifically Monsanto, now a part of Bayer—would harass or sue innocent farmers for patent violations if GMO seeds accidentally blew into their fields. Others believe pollen from GMO crops on neighboring farms will compromise the certification of organic farmers. Others came to believe that GMO crops were responsible for farmer suicides in India, and also for sheep deaths.

Defenders of GMOs have shown that none of these specific charges is supported by credible evidence. Regarding the environmental concerns, GMO corn pollen can certainly kill monarch butterfly caterpillars in laboratory experiments, but studies conducted by the EPA revealed that under open field conditions the risk was "negligible." Regarding superweeds and superbugs, some weeds did develop resistance to Roundup, the chemical herbicide used with GMO soybeans, but chemical resistance to herbicides predates GMOs, and a modification was soon made in the soybeans matched to a different herbicide, to which the weeds had not developed resistance. Meanwhile, Bt crops allow farmers to protect against insects while using fewer chemical sprays, not more.

Nor are the various food safety risks alleged for GMOs backed by scientific evidence. In Britain in 1998, the media gave loud play to the results of a laboratory experiment in which GMO potatoes were fed to rats, supposedly with damaging health effects, but the Royal Society later issued a statement saying that it was wrong to conclude anything from the experiment due to flaws in its design, and scientists using a proper study design never replicated the results. A study done in Austria in 2008 purported to find lower reproduction rates among mice that had been fed with GMO corn, but when the Scientific Panel on Genetically Modified Organisms of the EU reviewed the study, it found calculation errors, inconsistencies in treating the data, and an error in the method of calculating numbers of young mice (per pair rather than per delivering pair). The panel said that this nullified any conclusions that might be drawn from the study. Then in 2012, a French study supposedly showed that rats were more likely to develop tumors if they ate genetically modified corn sprayed with weed killer, but the European Food Safety Agency challenged the study immediately, asserting it was "of insufficient scientific quality to be considered as valid for risk assessment." It turned out that the breed of rat used in the experiment was specifically designed for a propensity to develop tumors.

Do genetically engineered crops strengthen corporate control?

Many charges against GMOs are based on fears that they change traditional relationships to food by weakening individual control and strengthening corporate control. Some aspects of this charge are easy to reject. For example, the widely held belief that GMOs have sterile seeds is simply false. GMO seeds do not contain so-called "terminator" genes; they are just as easy to replicate as non-GMO seeds. Indeed, the technology was spread on one occasion by farmers who got the seeds, took them across a border (from Argentina into Brazil), and then started planting, harvesting, and replanting them without official permission.

The fear that corporations will use patents on GMO seeds to gain excessive control is also an exaggeration. In most developing countries this is hardly a risk, because intellectual property laws in these countries usually do not permit the patenting of seeds. In countries that do permit seed patents, such as the United States and Canada, biotechnology companies like Monsanto/Bayer have indeed gone to court to defend their patent rights, creating something new for farmers to deal with. Yet nearly all commercial farmers in the United States and Canada have been more than willing to purchase GMO seeds every year rather than violate patents by harvesting and replanting them. This is because the purchased seeds will be of higher quality and will deliver cost savings that more than offset the price.

GMO critics frequently cite the case of a Canadian canola farmer named Percy Schmeiser, who in 1999 was sued by Monsanto for planting patented Roundup Ready canola seeds without a license. When it was shown that 50–95 percent of the canola in Schmeiser's field contained Monsanto's gene, he was unable to convince the Canadian Supreme Court that this many patented seeds had blown in from the road, and he lost the case. Schmeiser then countersued Monsanto for libel, trespass, and the contamination of his fields, but he lost that case too. Monsanto/Bayer does use aggressive legal tactics against those suspected of intentional patent infringement, but the company does not have a record of going to court over trace amounts of GMOs introduced accidentally or through cross-pollination.

The danger that accidental cross-pollination could lead to the decertification of organic farmers is also mostly imagined. The simple presence of detectable GMO material in a crop does not constitute a violation of the national organic standard in the United States. As long as the grower has not intentionally planted GMO seed, organic certification cannot be revoked.

A more legitimate concern in the United States, at the outset, was that GMO foods were sold in the market without an identifying label, whereas in most other advanced industrial countries, and in many developing countries as well, labels are legally mandated. Opinion research consistently showed that a strong majority of Americans wanted mandatory labels on GMOs, but the FDA said it had no authority to require labels so long as the genetic engineering process had introduced nothing significant for human health or safety. Then in 2012 a California ballot issue named Proposition 37 to mandate labels on GMO foods was launched with strong popular support. It failed by a narrow margin after a number of food and biotechnology companies (led by Monsanto, Kraft Foods, PepsiCo, and Coca-Cola) waged a $46 million public campaign in opposition. Supporters of mandatory labeling vowed to try again in other states, and in 2014 they finally succeeded in Vermont. To avoid the nightmare of a patchwork of different labeling requirements in many different states, the food companies then asked their friends in Congress to enact a weak, non-threatening national labeling law that would preempt any state laws—such as Vermont's law—that were stronger. Congress passed this weak law in 2016, one the food companies knew they could live with. This is because it used the term "bioengineered" rather than genetically engineered or GMO, because it did not apply to foods derived from GMOs without detectable transgenic material (e.g., soybean oil), and because the label could take the form of a QR code. The new law came into effect January 1, 2022. Most consumers didn't notice.

Are GMO foods and crops safe?

When GMO foods and crops were first placed on the market in the 1990s, some scientific bodies—for example, the British Medical Association (BMA)—initially held back from expressing an official opinion on the new technology. By the early 2000s, however, all of the most important science academies around the world—including the BMA—had concluded that there was no evidence of any new risk to human health or the environment from any of the GMO foods or crops that had been placed on the market up to that point.

This remains the official position of the BMA, the Royal Society in London, the French Academy of Sciences, and the German Academies of Science and Humanities. It is also the official position of the International Council for Science (ICSU), the Organisation for Economic Co-operation and Development (OECD) in Paris, the World Health Organization (WHO), and the Food and Agriculture Organization (FAO) of the UN. In 2010, the Research Directorate of the EU itself produced a report that went so far as to state that "biotechnology, and in particular GMOs, are not per se more risky than e.g. conventional plant breeding technologies." A 2016 committee at the National Academies of Science in the United States examined more than 900 research studies and stated the following: "The committee carefully searched all available research studies for persuasive evidence of adverse health effects directly attributable to consumption of foods derived from GE crops but found none."

Many skeptics are not persuaded by this absence of credible scientific evidence of new risks. They invoke a precautionary slogan, "Absence of evidence is not the same thing as evidence of absence." GMO defenders respond that if you spend more than two decades looking for evidence of a new risk and fail to find it, that may not be proof of absence (because nobody can prove a negative), but it should count as evidence of absence.

At a deeper psychological level, many skeptics resist GMO foods and crops not because of new risks, but because new benefits for consumers are largely absent. The first generation of GMO crops to come on the market helped farmers control weeds and insects at lower cost, but these GMOs did not provide a tangible direct benefit to food consumers. GMO maize and GMO soybeans did not look any better, taste any better, or nourish any better, and they did not make the processed foods that contained GMO ingredients noticeably cheaper in Europe or the United States. In the absence of a visible direct benefit, ordinary consumers saw nothing to lose from a highly precautionary stance. Consistent with this explanation is the fact that consumers—even in Europe—have not expressed any opposition to the use of genetic engineering in medical drugs, because from these products they do get direct benefits. These drugs can bring genuine risks, as documented in clinical trials, but because they also bring tangible direct benefits there is little or no popular resistance.

Could genetically engineered crops provide benefits to small farmers in developing countries?

They already have done so for small cotton farmers in China and India. China began planting GMO cotton in 1997, and by 2010 roughly 7 million small and resource-poor farmers were growing the crop, with average income gains estimated by

Clive James, from the International Service for the Acquisition of Agri-biotech Applications, at $220 per hectare. India has also done well with GMO cotton. One 2009 study by German-based economists Prakash Sadashivappa and Matin Qaim showed that in India farmers who adopted GMO cotton were able to reduce pesticide sprays by an average of 40 percent and realized yield gains of 30–40 percent, generating increased profits of roughly $60 per acre, even when the higher cost of the seed is taken into account. GMO cotton first became legal to plant in India in 2002, and within 10 years, more than 85 percent of cotton planted in India was GMO. More recently, 94 percent of India's cotton has been GMO.

Given this strong farmer support, it is anomalous that so many activist groups have claimed GMO cotton failed in India, so badly as to drive farmers to commit suicide. When the International Food Policy Research Institute investigated these claims in 2008, it found that rates of suicide among Indian farmers had not increased following the introduction of GMO cotton in 2002, and it confirmed that there would be no reason to expect such an increase, given the benefit to farmers that the technology was providing.

Beyond Bt cotton, it is more difficult to establish the benefits that GMOs might provide to small farmers in the developing world, mostly because it is not yet legal for most farmers in developing countries to plant any GMOs. Most national governments in the developing world decided to follow the European example by setting in place demanding and highly precautionary regulations governing GMOs. Some did this in the belief that European practices were the best practices (this was particularly the case for African countries with close post-colonial ties to Europe), while others were persuaded by activist NGOs that the technology was genuinely dangerous, or a commercial export risk in European markets.

These same NGOs had earlier promoted the negotiation of an international agreement—the 2000 Cartagena Protocol—governing the import and export of living GMOs (called

LMOs). This agreement was modeled after the 1989 Basel Convention on the Control of Transboundary Movements of Hazardous Wastes, an indication of how suspicious the authors of the protocol were toward agricultural biotechnology. The UN Environment Programme (UNEP) was given the lead in helping poor countries to implement the Cartagena Protocol, and it encouraged a European-style precautionary approach.

Critics of GMOs complained originally that the technology would be of little value to the developing world because most of the GMO traits on the market (like herbicide tolerance and insect resistance) were developed in corporate labs and then transferred into crops like soybeans or yellow maize grown by large commercial farmers in rich temperate zone countries. Because the seeds had been developed by private companies, they would be too expensive for poor farmers to afford. However, when Golden Rice was developed in 2000 by a noncorporate laboratory partly funded by the EU itself, and then offered to the developing world free of charge for humanitarian purposes, critics attacked it anyway, simply because it was a GMO. This new rice technology was developed specifically for poor tropical countries, to help reduce vitamin A deficiencies that cause some 250,000 children to go blind each year. Thanks to continuing hostility from critics and tight regulations even on the conduct of confined field trials in poor countries, Golden Rice was not approved for cultivation anywhere prior to 2021, when it finally got technical approval in the Philippines. In 2013, a UK environmentalist named Mark Lynas, who had helped launch the anti-GMO movement in the 1990s, took the unusual step of apologizing for his activism. Reversing his original views, he now described GMOs as a "desperately-needed agricultural innovation" that was being "strangled by a suffocating avalanche of regulations which are not based on any rational scientific assessment of risk."

Are CRISPR crops GMOs?

Modern biotechnology continues to provide new ways to modify the genetics of plants and animals. One new technique, which became the "scientific breakthrough of the year" in 2015, was genome editing, which can turn off individual plant and animal genes, or amplify their expression, without bringing in any "foreign DNA" from an unrelated species. The most popular of these genome editing techniques was named Clustered Regularly Interspaced Short Palindromic Repeats, or CRISPR. Diverse teams of scientists working in Europe, Canada, California, and Massachusetts got credit for the breakthrough.

CRISPR appears to promise even more rapid improvement in crop and animal genetics, and also in human medicine, compared to transgenic GMOs, because it is faster, cheaper, and even more precise. It also seemed likely, at first, that CRISPR crops would not trigger as many fears as GMOs, because most would contain no "foreign DNA." Gene editing closely resembled what happens when cells commonly undergo natural mutations, and the use of mutations to breed new crops has never triggered a "GMO" classification, even in Europe. Moreover, gene editing had been developed by scientists based in universities and nonprofit institutes, as opposed to corporate labs. A number of countries including the United States, Canada, and Sweden quickly announced they would not consider CRISPR crops GMOs for regulatory purposes.

Yet in 2018 the European Court of Justice, the supreme court for the entire EU, ruled that genome-edited crops, including CRISPR crops, should be regulated as GMOs, and thus be subject to the same labeling and tracing rules that were keeping GMOs out of farm fields and supermarkets in Europe. The court said gene-editing methods were not like mutation breeding because they lacked a long history of safe use (the same could have been said for Edison's light bulb when first invented). This court ruling hit European crop scientists hard.

One researcher at the Heinrich Heine University in Germany predicted it would be "the death blow for plant biotech in Europe."

Other governments around the world will now have to decide whether to follow Europe's highly precautionary approach to genome-edited foods, or follow the United States by allowing this new genetic alteration method to go forward. As of 2022, a majority were following the United States. Assuming CRISPR isn't the last breakthrough we will see in agricultural biotechnology, more regulatory struggles of this kind can be expected in the future.

14

WHO GOVERNS THE WORLD
FOOD SYSTEM?

Is there a single world food system?

Our so-called world food system is best understood as a collection of many distinct national food systems, increasingly connected by trade and international investment but not centrally controlled or governed. A significant share of the world's food does enter international trade. In 2019, the value of all food imports around the world was $1.4 trillion, making up a sizable portion of total global agricultural production (valued by FAO that year at $3.9 trillion). Yet food is still mostly produced and consumed within separately governed nation-states. We do not yet have a single, fully integrated world food market, and the international trade that takes place is not under any central control. One possible advantage of this fragmentation and decentralization is that no one political authority can disrupt the whole system. The disadvantage is that when international disruptions do occur, no single individual or institution is fully empowered to respond.

Despite increased globalization, most food around the world continues to be grown, harvested, processed, retailed, and consumed entirely within the borders of individual countries. Ninety percent of processed foods are never traded, along with 73 percent of wheat and 90 percent of rice. This pattern persists, despite the modern era of lower transport costs, because most countries do not want to depend on other countries for their basic food supply, so they have set in place policies intended to preserve independence and self-sufficiency. National governments remain the dominant actors in food and farming. They are in a position to take this leading role because of the exclusive legal jurisdiction they are entitled to enforce, as sovereign nations, over farms and food markets within their borders. The differing policies that national governments pursue can generate dramatically different food outcomes. For example, compare food circumstances today in Haiti and the Dominican Republic. These two states cohabit the same small Caribbean island, yet in poorly governed Haiti 47 percent of all citizens are undernourished, versus just 6.7 percent in the better-governed Dominican Republic. Or consider North and South Korea, states that share not just a common peninsula but also a common history, language, and national culture. Because the government of South Korea has governed its national economy and its national food system with conspicuous competence over the past half-century, chronic undernutrition has virtually disappeared. Because North Korea has not governed its economy and food system well, 42 percent of its citizens remain undernourished, and a million or more citizens died there not long ago in a devastating famine.

The dominating importance of national government policy in shaping food outcomes is also illustrated by the case of China. When China adopted an unwise food policy during Mao's Great Leap Forward, eliminating private markets and taking control of land away from farmers, the result was a famine in which 30 million people died between 1959 and 1961. When Mao's successor, Deng Xiaoping, introduced a new "household responsibility system" after 1978, reviving food marketing and peasant control over land, food production and income growth revived, and by 2002 the number of rural Chinese living in hunger and poverty had fallen by 89 percent.

How do national governments exercise control?

The policy instruments used by governments to shape food and farming systems differ between rich and poor countries. In rich countries, farmers often receive generous income subsidies and tax credits, plus protective trade restrictions at the border. It is not unusual to find a significant share of total farm income dependent on public policy (37 percent in Japan, in 2021). Off the farm, food systems in rich countries are heavily shaped by national tax and competition policies (e.g., antitrust) and increasingly by stronger regulations for food safety and environmental protection.

In poor countries, state interventions in the agricultural production and marketing sector can be just as powerful, but they are less likely to be farmer-friendly. In developing Asia, the centralized regulation of river valley irrigation systems has long given states an instrument to control farming. National programs governing the ownership and distribution of agricultural land (including periodic efforts at redistribution under the slogan of "land reform") are also a powerful governmental prerogative. State subsidies for fertilizers, pesticides, and electricity for irrigation pumps continue to play a system-shaping role. Countries like India operate state-run marketing systems to make staple foods available to the poor at a lower price, through (mostly urban) "fair price shops."

In much of Africa, state-controlled production and marketing systems that were originally created under colonial rule have continued to function as state-owned seed or chemical companies, or as "parastatal" marketing institutions granted near-monopoly rights by the government. The agricultural sectors in these African countries are more open to import competition and foreign direct investment than in the past, but private investment has lagged due to government restrictions, lagging government investments in infrastructure, and the failure of many governments to reduce official corruption and protect private property.

Which are the most important international organizations in the food and farming sector?

Above the level of the nation-state, the UN system includes organizations that can look like "global governance" institutions, but they usually have little influence over core activities within food and farming sectors.

For example, when food prices on the international market spiked in 2008, the secretary-general of the UN set up a high-level task force on the global food security crisis to produce an "action plan" prescribing an appropriate response. This gave an impression that the UN was taking charge, but in fact no new funding or authority was granted to the UN for this purpose, so the high-level task force had no measurable impact on either food production or consumption, and it posed no threat to national governmental control. Something similar had happened during the earlier world food crisis of 1974, when the UN response was to create a largely toothless committee on world food security.

The more significant reactions to the 2008 price spike came not from the UN system but from the national governments of the major economic powers, acting either alone or in concert. These governments assemble for periodic summit meetings as the Group of 8 (G8) and the Group of 20 (G20). The G20 was established in 1999 in the wake of the East Asian financial crisis as a means to broaden international consultations beyond the smaller G8 cluster of advanced industrial states. The G8 became the G7 when Russia withdrew in 2017. The G20 includes emerging and transitional economic powers such as Brazil, China, India, Indonesia, South Africa, and Turkey. Both the G7 and the G20 meet on a regular basis at the head of state (or "summit") level, and in these settings significant national policy changes or resource commitments can be pursued. After the price spike of 2008, it was at a G8 summit meeting, in July 2009, that the world's leading powers concluded the financially significant L'Aquila pledge to increase agricultural development assistance.

The purpose of such G7 and G20 meetings is to facilitate co-operation among nation-states, not to replace or override those states. For example, when President Nicolas Sarkozy of France attempted in 2011 to use his temporary chairmanship of a G20 Summit to promote reforms in commodity futures trading, biofuels, and export policies, he was effectively blocked from this goal by the other major economic powers, including the United States, the UK, Brazil, and Russia.

Some prominent international organizations also function as settings for national governments to negotiate, which once again empowers rather than controls those governments. One example is the World Trade Organization (WTO), originally created as the General Agreement on Tariffs and Trade (GATT) at an international conference in Bretton Woods, New Hampshire, in 1944. The WTO is headquartered in Geneva, where it provides a setting for national governments to negotiate agreements on trade, including agricultural trade. The WTO even has a Dispute Settlement Body (DSB) to adjudicate claims from member governments regarding the non-compliance of others with these international agreements. In the past, both the cotton policies of the United States and the sugar and GMO policies of the EU have triggered successful complaints of this kind. Deliberations within the DSB can draw on the findings of one other international institution, the Codex Alimentarius ("food code") Commission in Rome, a body created by the UN in 1963 to develop common global standards for safe food products and fair food trade practices. Because Codex operates by consensus, global standards tend not to be finalized in controversial areas such as GMOs.

The International Monetary Fund (IMF) and the World Bank are two other international institutions created at Bretton Woods in 1944. They are largely funded by wealthy country governments and are empowered to make sizable loans to governments in developing countries, particularly those facing financial crises or struggling to create a policy environment to support sustained economic growth. The lending conditions imposed by the IMF traditionally included market deregulation and an end to inflationary fiscal and monetary policies. The World Bank in the 1960s and 1970s became a significant source of lending for investments in agricultural development, but following the success of the green revolution it cut lending to agriculture and moved on to other concerns. When world food prices spiked in 2008, the World Bank president, Robert Zoellick, vowed to revive work in the area of agricultural development, and new loans were made, particularly to Africa. The World Bank also became home to the new Global Agriculture and Food Security Program, created in 2009 at the insistence of the G20, but national governments fell short in the resources contributed to this fund. The IMF and the World Bank are both headquartered in Washington, DC, and have traditionally embraced a so-called Washington Consensus that emphasizes the role of free markets and private investments, as opposed to state planning, market controls, and government subsidies.

Within the food and agricultural sectors, the UN system has four "Rome institutions": Codex Alimentarius, IFAD, WFP, and FAO. The youngest of these is the International Fund for Agricultural Development (IFAD), established in 1977 to finance agricultural development projects focused specifically on hunger reduction and rural poverty alleviation. The IFAD is less constrained by the Washington Consensus than either the IMF or the World Bank, but at the same time it has fewer lending resources. A second Rome organization, the UN World Food Programme (WFP), was established in 1961 to manage the delivery of humanitarian food assistance to poor countries and refugee populations. Individual donor governments are still the source of nearly all international food aid, but more than half is now channeled to its destination by the WFP.

The oldest and most prominent Rome-based UN institution is the Food and Agriculture Organization (FAO). Founded in 1945, the FAO devotes much of its energy to gathering, studying, and distributing information about food and farming around the world. It also provides a forum for nations to meet to set goals, share expertise, and seek agreement on agricultural policy. At the FAO, agricultural ministries from member governments are often in the lead, so this organization has traditionally placed greater emphasis on food production and the prosperity of farmers than on the nutrition of consumers. Within the UN system, nutrition issues were traditionally handled by the World Health Organization.

In the area of agricultural research and technology development, the most important international institution is the Consultative Group on International Agricultural Research (CGIAR), a network of research centers created in 1971 and chaired by the World Bank. The CGIAR eventually expanded into a network of 15 separate international centers (later reduced to 14), primarily located in the developing world and funded by government donors and private foundations, plus the World Bank. These centers have attempted to extend the legacy of the original green revolution of the 1960s and 1970s by using science to develop improved seeds and more productive and sustainable farming methods in order to help farmers in the developing world.

What has limited the influence of international organizations?

The political influence of these international food and agricultural institutions has differed case by case. In the 1980s and 1990s, the WTO achieved measurable success by hosting the Uruguay Round of negotiations that locked in some reductions in the rich country farm subsidy policies that were distorting trade. The Agreement on Agriculture that emerged from these negotiations in 1993 required industrial countries to convert nontariff agricultural border protections to tariffs, instruments that allow important price signals to operate. The agreement imposed no restriction on direct cash payments to farmers, so long as those payments were decoupled from production incentives. The agreement also prohibited direct export subsidies, but it did nothing to prevent governments from disrupting markets through export bans, which emerged as a larger short-run concern at the time of the 2008 price spike, and then returned as an issue in 2022 when the war in Ukraine broke out.

Following its partly successful Uruguay Round effort, the WTO launched a new Doha Round in 2001, but these negotiations were suspended without any result seven years later, in part because of disagreements between the United States and India over exceptions to the agreed disciplines on import restrictions. In 2015 a WTO ministerial session in Nairobi did reach a useful agreement to limit export subsidies, but by then it was clear that international agricultural trade was distorted more by periodic export bans, not export subsidies.

Even when governments voluntarily accept policy restraints under the WTO, they sometimes fail to comply. For example, in 2005, the United States was told by the DSB that elements of its cotton subsidy program were illegal under the 1993 Agreement on Agriculture, but the United States refused either to change its policies adequately or to pay compensation. In 2008, the US Congress even passed a new farm bill explicitly preserving some of the WTO-illegal policies. When Brazil eventually threatened retaliation in 2010, the United States responded not by changing its cotton policy but instead by offering compensation payments to cotton growers in Brazil. The final outcome was ironic: US taxpayers began paying for cotton subsidies in two countries rather than just one.

The IMF and the World Bank had considerable influence over food and farming in the 1980s and 1990s, when they used stabilization agreements, investment loans, and "structural adjustment" loans to shape the price and market environment for farmers in poor developing countries. Yet the policy changes they hoped to induce were sometimes small or just temporary. In 1994, the World Bank completed a study of 29 governments in Sub-Saharan Africa that had undergone structural adjustment and found 17 of those 29 had indeed reduced the overall tax burden they placed on farming, but some, because of persistently overvalued exchange rates, had nonetheless increased that burden. Only 4 of the 29 had eliminated parastatal marketing boards for major export crops, and none of the 29 had set in place both agricultural and macroeconomic policies measuring up to World Bank standards. Later, the International Food Policy Research Institute found that many of the reforms undertaken in response to World Bank pressures were reversed when conditions changed or in response to external shocks.

The World Bank gave away much of its influence over global agriculture beginning in the 1980s, when it began to cut the total value of its lending in that sector. Between 1978 and 2006, the agricultural share of World Bank lending fell from 30 percent to only 8 percent. In 2005, the World Bank president, Paul Wolfowitz, even admitted in an offhand comment, "My institution's largely gotten out of the business of agriculture." To explain this withdrawal of lending for agriculture, officials at the World Bank claimed it was the borrowing country governments who had changed their priorities, but priorities at the Bank had changed as well. Lending for policy change (called "structural adjustment") was crowding out lending for actual investments in development.

Of the three Rome-based UN food organizations, the WFP and IFAD are frequently praised for their work. The WFP has a proven record of preventing famine, as in the case of the 1991–1992 and 2001–2002 droughts in southern Africa. Although the WFP failed to prevent a famine in southern Somalia in 2011, the reason was blocked access due to the intransigence of an armed jihadist militia group, al-Shabaab. WFP was awarded the Nobel Peace Prize in 2020, in recognition of the assistance it had provided in the previous year to nearly 100 million people facing hunger and acute food insecurity in 88 countries around the world.

FAO's reputation for taking effective action is not as strong. In fact, it was international frustration with the FAO during the world food crisis of the 1970s that led to the creation of the IFAD in 1977. The data collection activities of the FAO are highly regarded, and in some niche areas (e.g., the integrated management of crop pests, or IPM), FAO technical advice can be world class, but its operations are heavily dominated by an oversized central bureaucracy. It has also been burdened by lethargic leadership over the years, from officials chosen by their political friends, despite deficits in their professional expertise or engagement, a pattern sometimes encountered in other UN's special agencies as well. Looking at the budget of the FAO, more than half has usually been spent on headquarters operations within the city of Rome, not in the developing world.

In the area of internationally funded agricultural research, the multiple centers of the CGIAR have had a four-decade history of success in developing useful new farm technologies for the developing world. The improved rice varieties originally developed by the International Rice Research Institute have now been released in more than 77 countries, allowing the world to more than double total rice production since 1965. Two-thirds of the developing world's total area planted to wheat is now planted to varieties that contain improvements developed by the CGIAR's International Maize and Wheat Improvement Center. Nevertheless, the CGIAR has struggled since the 1990s to maintain adequate donor funding, due partly to complacency among those who thought the world's food production problems had already been solved, plus hostility from others who reject a science-forward green revolution approach. The CGIAR's approach is not ideal in every respect; too much crop science is conducted under artificial conditions at the centers, without adequate testing in actual farmers' fields, and too often the new technologies developed never reach the intended beneficiaries. The successful uptake of improved methods by poor farmers almost always requires partnership with strong research and extension institutions at the national level, and too often in recent years these also have been underfunded.

Do multinational corporations control the world food system?

Some scholars and activists assert that large corporations do exercise international control, through monopoly positions in key markets and the direct investments they make across borders, plus the corrupting influence they sometimes exercise over individual national governments. Intergovernmental organizations like the WTO, the IMF, and the World Bank are described by these critics as little more than global agents created to reinforce this corporate control.

Assertions of corporate monopoly in the food sector usually begin with claims that 70 percent of international grain trade goes through the hands of just four private companies: Archer Daniels Midland, Bunge, Cargill, and Louis Dreyfus—known collectively as the ABCD traders. A 2012 study commissioned by the NGO Oxfam described the control of these companies as far-reaching:

> Through their roles in biofuels investment, large-scale land acquisition, and the financialization of agricultural commodity markets, the ABCDs are at the forefront of the transformation that is determining where money in agriculture is invested, where agricultural production is located, where the produce is shipped, and how the world's population shares (or fails to share) the bounty of each harvest.

When considering such assessments, it is important to remember that less than 30 percent of world grain production ever enters international trade, so the control available to companies specializing in that trade will automatically be limited. Also, despite the market concentration these four trading companies still compete with each other for customers, and they purchase what they sell at prices set in open and publicly regulated commodity futures markets. Finally, those alleging corporate control over grain markets seldom make a consistent argument regarding the impact of that control. Some say that the companies conspire to make international grain prices artificially low ("dumping" surplus production into poor countries), while others blame the companies for driving grain prices artificially high. In reality, grain-trading companies make money whether international prices are high or low. They do so by knowing the needs of their customers and skillfully responding to price changes rather than by controlling those changes.

The alleged dominance of these private ABCD companies is now directly challenged in any case by a state-controlled Chinese company, COFCO International, which imports foodstuffs into China and sells to more than 50 countries, especially in Europe, the Black Sea, and Latin America. By 2018, COFCO International was moving 105 million tons of grain, oilseeds, and sugar a year, a tonnage roughly equal to America's entire soybean crop.

Critics have also asserted that corporate agribusiness investments in regions such as Africa have led to the marginalization of poor subsistence crop farmers. This ignores the fact that Africa, since decolonization, has attracted very little investment from private agribusiness firms. The companies take little interest in African farmers because most are too poor to purchase farm equipment and seeds, or to produce a marketable surplus. More than 60 percent of all Africans work in the agricultural sector, yet only 5 percent of foreign direct investment in Africa goes to this sector, and foreign investments in Africa are minuscule to begin with, adding up to just 4 percent of the total flow of global foreign investment. The danger is not that MNCs will control poor farmers in Africa, but instead that they will continue to ignore them.

Corporate control is also said to derive from seed patents, such as those registered by companies like Monsanto (now Bayer). One important limitation to this argument is that in most countries, especially developing countries, national laws do not allow patent claims on seeds. In addition, many developing world farmers buy no seeds at all, let alone patented seeds. In the Indian Punjab, 74 percent of farmers still plant their own saved seeds, and when Indian farmers do buy seeds, they have 500 private Indian seed companies to turn to, not just multinationals like DuPont Pioneer or Bayer/Monsanto. Meanwhile, national biosafety regulations plus consumer resistance have tightly restricted the planting of patented seeds, even in those rich countries that allow patents. As of 2022 there were still no patented GMO wheat or rice seeds on the market anywhere, not even in the United States.

Corporate control over seed markets is also weakened by competition. For example, when Monsanto tried to market a new corn seed variety called "Smartstax" in 2010, it overpriced the product and lost market shares to a competitor seed company, DuPont Pioneer (now named Corteva). In the end, Monsanto had to reduce its price premium by 67 percent in order to win back customers, and even then it failed to recover market share.

The allegation that private food and agribusiness companies exercise influence over national governments by paying bribes does have some foundation. In one sensational exposé in 2012, investigators learned that a subsidiary of Walmart in Mexico had bribed local and national officials to speed the building of 19 large new stores, sometimes without construction permits. In some cases, Walmart paid nearly a million dollars in bribes per store. In an earlier case, Monsanto was required to pay a $1.5 million fine (to the US Justice Department) for having bribed an Indonesian official in 2002, to get around an environmental impact study on its cotton seeds. In this case, however, the bribe was unsuccessful because the requirement for the study was never waived, and Monsanto's cotton seeds never became legal to plant. Even in countries where bribery is common, then, the bribe may not always result in corporate control.

How much power do non-governmental organizations have?

International non-governmental organizations (NGOs) are influential players within food and farming sectors, especially in the developing world. Some development NGOs work almost exclusively through projects on the ground. For example, Heifer International operates projects in 21 different countries to promote food self-reliance through gifts of livestock plus training. Other NGOs work almost exclusively through social mobilization and advocacy. One example is La Via Campesina (LVC), an organization founded in 1986 to oppose corporate globalization, and to promote "food sovereignty" for small farmers. LVC is a network of local and national organizations in 70 different countries. Greenpeace, an environmental advocacy organization based in Amsterdam, also campaigns against globalization and agribusiness, particularly against genetically engineered crops. Greenpeace claims 3 million supporters worldwide. Consumers International, a global federation of more than 250 advocacy organizations in 120 different countries, promotes consumer food safety.

In the areas such as food safety and farm technology, NGO criticism sometimes succeeds in exposing and even blocking suspect corporate actions. In the 1970s, a network of NGOs accused Nestlé of promoting infant formula products through unethical methods, such as giving away free samples in maternity wards. An NGO-led boycott of Nestlé products, driven by the inflammatory slogan "Nestlé Kills Babies," eventually led to a new International Code of Marketing of Breast-milk Substitutes, which Nestlé pledged to follow in 1984. Also in the 1980s, an international NGO advocacy campaign led by the Pesticides Action Network managed to produce an International Code of Conduct on the Distribution and Use of Pesticide, and later a binding international agreement named the Rotterdam Convention. In the 1990s, European-based NGOs spread alarms about genetically engineered crops that led in a few years to a virtual ban on the planting of those crops in Europe and to regulatory blockage in much of the rest of the world as well. In 2013, an activist from the UK who had participated in these anti-GMO campaigns, but who later changed his mind about the technology and apologized, admitted, "This was the most successful campaign I have ever been involved in."

Not all advocacy NGOs work to block things. In the area of food security, some groups like Bread for the World use information and advocacy campaigns to promote food aid and agricultural development. Others, like Oxfam, combine research and policy advocacy with actual development projects on the ground (Oxfam calls itself a "do tank"). Still others, like Catholic Relief Services, work almost exclusively delivering humanitarian relief. In the area of agricultural development, however, there are limits to what NGOs from the outside can accomplish on their own. They deliver excellent training and services but are less able to provide the expensive infrastructure investments in roads, electricity, irrigation, and in agricultural research that are needed in many of the poorest countries. National governments and donor agencies with taxpayer-derived resources must take the lead here.

International NGOs in food and agriculture are typically funded and headquartered in rich countries, so they tend to export the concerns of rich countries into the developing world. In areas such as health and human rights, this is usually appropriate, but in the area of agricultural technology the concerns of the rich are not always well matched to the needs of the poor. Farm chemical use is clearly excessive in Europe and North America, but in most of Africa fertilizer use is too low, and needs to be increased. When European or American

NGOs carry their campaigns against chemical fertilizer into Africa, they can push local policy in the wrong direction.

What is the role of private foundations?

Independently endowed philanthropic foundations such as the Rockefeller Foundation and the Ford Foundation played an essential role in launching Asia's original green revolution in the 1960s and 1970s. More recently it has been the Bill and Melinda Gates Foundation that has done the most to promote the green revolution cause.

The Ford Foundation, with roughly $12 billion in assets, is an important New York–based institution that provided early support to the green revolution in Asia but later moved away from promoting science-dependent approaches to farming. Although the Rockefeller Foundation had assets only one-half the size of Ford, it was more important in launching the green revolution and it continued to stress the importance of agricultural science in developing countries long after Ford drifted away from that cause. Then, in 2006, the Bill and Melinda Gates Foundation, which had $37 billion in assets at the time, moved decisively into grant-making in agricultural development (adopting Rockefeller as a junior partner), beginning with a $150 million joint venture called the Alliance for a Green Revolution in Africa (AGRA), chaired by former UN secretary-general Kofi Annan. This initiative centered on an effort to improve the varieties of seed available to small farmers for staple food crops in Africa. By 2012, the Gates Foundation had made grants for agricultural development totaling more than $2 billion.

By supporting seed markets, new agricultural science, and a "green revolution," the Gates Foundation knew that it would be inviting criticism from those in the NGO community who mistrusted this approach. Soon after the foundation announced its new effort, an NGO based in the United States named Food First warned that Bill and Melinda Gates were "naïve about the causes of hunger" and that their efforts would only provide "higher profits for the seed and fertilizer industries, negligible impacts on total food production and worsening exclusion and marginalization in the countryside." Others in the philanthropic community who were timid about facing hostile NGO criticism continued to shrink away from promoting science-based, market-oriented agricultural development.

Such differences took center stage in 2021 when the UN secretary-general, António Guterres, convened a Food Systems Summit in New York. A group of more than 500 NGOs ("civil society organizations" is the label they prefer) objected to the meeting and stayed away because Guterres had formed a "strategic partnership" with the World Economic Forum, an organization famous for hosting meetings of corporate leaders every year in Davos, Switzerland. They also objected because Guterres had announced that his special envoy to lead the summit would be Dr. Agnes Kalibata, a Rwandan agricultural scientist and president of AGRA, which the NGOs accused of promoting the interests of agribusiness. The NGOs wanted the meeting to promote agroecology, not the green revolution.

Although the secretary-general got caught on this occasion in a conflict between civil society NGOs, philanthropic foundations, and multinational corporations, the impacts were minimal. The summit was never going to be capable of meeting its stated goal of "food system transformation." As has been shown, the power to transform food systems rests primarily in the hands of national governments within their own sovereign borders at home, not in the hands of UN bureaucrats, NGOs, philanthropists, or even multinational corporations at a meeting in New York.

15

THE FUTURE OF FOOD POLITICS

Is the world food system being transformed by crisis?

On repeated occasions in the recent past it seemed that the world food system was facing a transformational crisis. Rapid population growth in the 1960s convinced many that widespread famines were inevitable, and when international grain prices spiked in the 1970s some thought that dark prediction was coming true. Thanks to adequate investments in agricultural productivity, that calamity was avoided. When international prices spiked again in 2008, mostly due to a combination of inflationary monetary policies and national export bans, journalists said it would be "the end of cheap food," but that didn't happen either. Then in 2022, when the Ukraine war, more inflationary policies, and another round of export bans briefly spiked prices once again, many jumped to a conclusion that our food system lacked resilience and needed to be urgently "transformed" to survive shocks like COVID, conflict, and climate change (called "the 3 Cs").

If we step back from this repeating pattern of short-term panic and dire predictions, the bigger food picture that emerges is one of considerable achievement. Despite continued population growth, the share of individuals in the developing world suffering from chronic undernourishment fell from 36 percent in 1970 to 20 percent in 1990, and then down to just 11 percent by 2017. What made this possible was a successful economic transformation, with large numbers of people managing to escape poverty. World Bank data show that the share of the world's population living in poverty fell from 42 percent in 1981 to just 8.6 percent by 2018. These more prosperous global citizens were able to get the larger quantities of food they wanted thanks to a parallel agricultural transformation: science was providing new farming tools that made possible the production of much more food on less land. In fact, total global land used for crops and pasture finally stopped increasing in 2001, according to FAO, and began to decline, even while food consumption remained rapidly on the rise.

Applications of modern science to farming have allowed large parts of the world to produce and deliver more food while using less land, water, energy, and fewer chemicals for every added bushel. We have called this a transition to "ecomodern" farming, made possible in part by the tools of precision agriculture. Farming in rich countries is using digital technology to become information-intensive rather than resource-intensive. This is a transition that needs to continue. In Sub-Saharan Africa, however, smallholder farming is still mostly premodern. The transition out of poverty and toward ecomodern farming has been lagging badly and needs a stronger political push.

Is obesity replacing hunger as the world's most serious food problem?

In terms of the numbers affected, yes. The World Health Organization currently estimates more than 1 billion people worldwide are obese, twice the 2008 number, and more than FAO's estimate of those who are chronically undernourished (between 702 million and 828 million in 2021). A global political response to this obesity crisis has only just begun to emerge. An organization named the World Obesity Federation (which created a World Obesity Day, every March 4) now raises money to promote understanding, prevention, and treatment of the condition, but effective prevention policies have proved difficult to implement.

While the world has learned over the years how to reduce hunger, primarily by promoting income growth while investing in more productive farming, it is still struggling to find acceptable policies to reduce obesity. In liberal societies these policies cannot be coercive, and should not increase stigma. In some countries prevention measures like taxes on sugary beverages and restrictions on advertising unhealthy foods to children have finally gained acceptance, but not yet in the United States. An easier path for America to follow may be one of acceptance and treatment, rather than prevention. This will be expensive, and it will work better for Americans with resources than for those without.

While obesity will deserve much more attention in the years ahead, there are good reasons for government policies in much of the world to remain focused on those who still consume too little food rather than too much, since those who are still undernourished have fewer options for self-help. Redefining the world's food problem as obesity *rather* than hunger would carry a significant ethical risk. In Sub-Saharan Africa today, only 5 percent of children under five are overweight, while 31 percent are stunted. In many villages in rural Africa and South Asia, undernutrition remains the dominant food-related concern, and it is one for which we have proven solutions, so there is no excuse for inaction.

In the future, will food and farming systems become more localized or more globalized?

Food and farming systems have been growing more specialized, and consequently less localized, for a long time now. The anthropologists Gretel and Pertti Pelto have described this process as a "fundamental, apparently unidirectional tendency in human history." Food and farming are similar to many other modern production and marketing systems in this regard.

They are being driven toward greater globalization by falling transportation costs, increasing income and consumption demands in previously poor countries, and political barriers to international investment and trade that are lower than in the past. Market competition drives all production systems to cut costs, which usually results in greater specialization, so over time individual production units shrink in number but grow in size, while products travel greater distances. Market volatility drives production units to reduce risks through formally structured or contracted business-to-business relationships, yet thanks to competition and continuing innovation, the prices offered to consumers usually decline over the long run. Between 1961 and 2010, the average real international price for cereals, meats, dairy, and sugar products actually declined by 40 percent. The real price of milk to American consumers fell 18 percent between 1995 and 2021 alone.

In the future, it is unlikely that today's rich countries will move back toward food systems based less on globalization and more on localization, or based less on specialization and more on diversification. Niche markets for locally grown foods will continue to expand as consumer purchasing power grows and preferences diversify, but a preponderance of consumers will continue to use the conventional market channels that can offer lower costs, greater convenience, and more choices year-round.

In the future, low- and middle-income countries will become less poor, more urban, and consequently more like today's rich countries in the ways they produce and consume food. Eating habits worldwide will continue to converge toward common sets of practices, including an increased reliance on foods purchased (electronically or in person) at supermarkets; increased consumption of packaged and processed foods, frozen foods, meat, eggs, and dairy products; and also year-round consumption of more nutritious fresh fruits and vegetables. One common feature in this convergence will be a wider range of affordable eating choices, both healthy and un-healthy. Different communities and different individuals will make their food choices in different ways, leading to highly divergent health and nutrition outcomes, as in the United States today, but the choices available will continue to expand for nearly all. Individual diets will continue to move away from being determined by national residence or cultural heritage. Conscious personal choice will play an ever-larger role; this will benefit those who are health-conscious, while possibly putting others at risk.

In the future, will the spread of more affluent eating habits destroy the natural environment?

The answer is yes, unless food production systems evolve even more rapidly toward less dependence on land, water, and chemical inputs for every pound of production, and toward reduced dependence on natural systems such as wild fisheries. Difficult debates will nonetheless continue over trusting modern science to move food production in this direction, and over who should be trusted with the science. The science-forward ecomodernists will disagree with the agroecologists who want food production systems to protect nature by imitating nature, or simply by producing less. Commercial farmers will see agroecology as unrewarding, and consumers will resist any loss of choice, so food and farming will continue to evolve in a science-forward direction, but perhaps not quickly enough to bring a halt to environmental destruction, given unabated climate change and continued population increases in vulnerable regions such as Africa.

Dietary austerity will be difficult to achieve without coercion, which is a pathway free societies should not wish to follow. Excessive consumption of ruminant animal products might be slowed through greater health-consciousness, a continuing substitution of poultry for beef, and through the development of more appealing plant-based or cell-grown substitutes for meat, dairy, and egg products. Continued investments in crop science, irrigation engineering, remote sensing, GPS positioning, AI, machine learning, and robotics can bring down the resource burden of food production. Industrial agriculture can become increasingly postindustrial: information-intensive rather than resource-intensive.

What will worry optimists is a continuing lag in the research investments needed to ensure that the pace of innovation will continue, especially within the less productive tropical farming systems of South Asia and Africa. All agricultural systems face highly localized challenges that can only be met through investments in local innovation. Inadequate external support for agricultural research in the poor countries of Africa, plus accelerating climate change, present a daunting challenge. The environmental price of failing to improve Africa's low-yield farming systems will be more trees felled, more soil nutrients mined, more fragile lands plowed and ruined, and more wildlife habitat destroyed to accommodate a relentless spread of low-yield farming, as population continues to increase.

The global spread of more affluent eating habits will directly threaten the world's wild ocean fisheries. Middle-class consumers in Asia will continue to demand more fish. China, the world's largest seafood consumer, continues to expand its long-range fishing fleet at a time when 87 percent of global fisheries are already considered fully exploited, overexploited, or depleted. This growing threat to wild fish populations can be reduced through the production of more "farmed" fish, both in and away from saltwater, but making aquaculture environmentally sustainable and politically acceptable is still an unsolved problem. Larger investments in research and innovation may provide answers, but the skeptics will balk, wishing instead that we could simply consume less.

In the future, will climate change become the dominant source of food system transformation?

Agricultural systems everywhere will be forced to adjust to climate change, which will bring higher temperatures, more extreme droughts and floods, and sea-level rise that will threaten low-lying coastal communities. Over the long run, food systems will be significantly transformed, but the changes are likely to be incremental rather than sudden or dramatic. High-income countries will have the time and resources to make relatively successful food system adaptations, at least over the next several decades. Low-income countries with fewer resources, especially those already struggling with high temperatures, water shortages, and weather extremes, will face far more difficult adjustments. One of these adjustments will be an accelerating migration of people from low-income to high-income regions. In Bangladesh, where one-third of the population lives along a low-lying coast, more than 13 million people, or nearly 10 percent of the population, may have to leave the country by 2050.

With adequate investment in agricultural R&D and irrigation infrastructures, high-income societies will be able to continue boosting farm productivity, at least in the short run. But climate change is already making this more difficult. One 2021 study from Stanford University found that total factor productivity in global farming would have grown 25 percent more than it actually did over the previous 60 years, if climate change had not already been under way.

In several different lower income regions, adjustments to climate change will grow increasingly difficult. In Africa, more than 50 percent of all individuals depend on rain-fed agriculture for their livelihoods. For coastal and island countries in Africa, sea-level rise will lead to coastal erosion and saltwater flooding, disrupting both crop farming and traditional fishing communities. The World Bank estimates that flooding from rivers bursting their banks due to intense rainfall, and coastal erosion due to sea-level rise, are now costing just four small countries in West Africa (Benin, Côte d'Ivoire, Senegal, and Togo) $3.8 billion and 13,000 deaths a year. In Ghana, coastal erosion has already turned fishing villages into islands.

In the water-stressed regions of the Middle East and North Africa, the International Food Policy Research Institute projects that by 2050 cereal crop yields will be 4.8 percent lower than would have been possible otherwise, due to climate change. In South Asia, where higher temperatures over the Himalaya mountains are causing glaciers to shrink, the river waters downstream that supply essential crop irrigation systems will flow in less manageable patterns, eventually shrinking as well. These glaciers have already lost more mass since 2000 than they lost in the entire 20th century. More extreme precipitation events are already damaging crops. In 2017 flash floods damaged about 220,000 hectares of rice in Bangladesh, and in the summer of 2022 abnormally heavy rains in Pakistan turned the Indus River valley into a vast lake, submerging one-third of the country, killing 1,600 people, and destroying 15 percent of the nation's rice crop.

In the future, will the politics of food remain contentious?

Yes, and in some ways it might become more contentious. In prosperous countries, political debates over farm policy are moving beyond traditional questions of material gain, such as who owns the land, or who gets the biggest crop subsidies. At issue now are contested values, such as what an ideal rural landscape should look like. Should farms be large-scale and specialized, or small-scale and diversified? What kind of farming works best to protect nature and slow climate change? Such questions will become more contentious as the number of people who actually make their living from farming continues to decline. Increasingly, it will mostly be non-farmers, without firsthand knowledge of crop and livestock production, who will set the terms of the debate. The questions will less often be about the productivity of farms, or the income of farmers, and more often about what kind of farming is humane, sustainable, and just.

At the consumption end, a similar transition will take place. As food becomes increasingly safe to eat, increasingly affordable, and abundant in endless variety year-round, the concerns of consumers will also move away from issues of cost or safety toward less material concerns, including those driven by ethics and culture.

In these realms of ethics and culture, advocates for the status quo always find themselves on the defensive. It is never enough for them to show that the present is better than the past. Average producers and consumers in the marketplace might be comfortable with the trends they see in today's food and farm systems, but cultural critics and opinion leaders will continue to imagine and promote more attractive, or seemingly more attractive, alternatives. One result will be a growing divergence between actual commercial outcomes and the stated preferences of cultural elites. As food systems become more globalized, leaders in this cultural marketplace may continue calling for a return to local food. As modern farms continue to specialize and grow in size, cultural leaders may continue to champion a return to smaller and more diversified farms.

Will it be possible, in the future, for one set of trends in the commercial arena to coexist with an opposing set of preferences in the cultural arena? It usually falls to political leaders to resolve such tensions, typically through efforts to please both sides. In the United States, government leaders—so far—have allowed food and farming systems to continue an evolution toward a larger scale, increased specialization, and more internationalization, so as to continue serving consumer demands for cost savings, variety, and convenience. Industry lobbies that favor these trends have continued to hold the upper hand, and most ordinary voters seem comfortable with these trends as well. Elected leaders have therefore decided, for now, not to use their tax and regulatory powers to force farming back toward a smaller, more local, more diverse, or less science-based model. They have concluded, for now, that voters and campaign contributors will punish any attempt to reduce the range of eating choices currently enjoyed by citizens, no matter how unhealthy some of those choices might be. This light-handed governmental approach has functioned well enough, so far, within America's political culture favoring personal liberty and individual choice.

In wealthy societies where a heavier government hand is permitted—such as Japan, or on the continent of Europe—leaders in the future might attempt stronger measures to preserve traditional agrarian landscapes, or to constrain unhealthy eating. But this will also be contentious. From the vantage point of today, we cannot be certain where a political equilibrium will settle in the end.

SUGGESTIONS FOR FURTHER READING

Food Production and Population Growth

Bailey, Ronald, and Marian L. Tupy, *Ten Global Trends Every Smart Person Should Know*. Washington, DC: CATO Institute, 2020.

Bremer, Jason. *Population and Food Security: Africa's Challenge*. Washington, DC: Population Reference Bureau, Policy Brief, 2012.

Conway, Gordon. *One Billion Hungry: Can We Feed the World?* Ithaca, NY: Cornell University Press, 2012.

Diamond, Jared. *Collapse: How Societies Choose to Fail or Succeed*. New York: Penguin, 2005.

Lappé, Frances Moore, and Joseph Collins. *Diet for a Small Planet*. New York: Ballantine Books, 1971.

Malthus, Thomas Robert. *An Essay on the Principle of Population*. Cambridge: Cambridge University Press, 1992.

Paddock, William, and Paul Paddock. *Famine, 1975! America's Decision: Who Will Survive?* Boston: Little, Brown, 1967.

Pinker, Steven. *Enlightenment Now: The Case for Reason, Science, Humanism, and Progress*. New York: Viking, 2018.

United Nations. *World Population Prospects 2022: Summary of Results*. New York: United Nations, 2022.

World Bank. *World Development Report 2008: Agriculture for Development*. Washington, DC: World Bank, 2007.

The Politics of International Food Prices

Barrett, Christopher B., ed. *Food Security and Sociopolitical Stability*. New York: Oxford, 2013.

Pardey, P. G., J. M. Alston, and R. R. Piggott, eds. *Agricultural R&D in the Developing World: Too Little, Too Late?* Washington, DC: International Food Policy Research Institute, 2006.

US Department of Agriculture, Economic Research Service. *International Food Security Assessment, 2022–32.* Outlook Report No. GFA-33, Agriculture and Trade Reports. Washington, DC: US Department of Agriculture, 2022.

The Politics of Chronic Hunger

Ahmed, Akhter U., Ruth Vargas Hill, Lisa C. Smith, Doris M. Wiesmann, and Tim Frankenberger. *The World's Most Deprived: Characteristics and Causes of Extreme Poverty and Hunger.* 2020 Discussion Paper 43. Washington, DC: International Food Policy Research Institute, 2007.

Food and Agriculture Organization of the United Nations. *State of Food and Nutrition Security in the World, 2022.* Rome: FAO, 2022. https:// www.fao.org/publications/sofi/2022/en.

Lipton, Michael. *Why Poor People Stay Poor: Urban Bias in World Development.* Cambridge, MA: Harvard University Press, 1977.

Resnick, Danielle, et al. *Global Hunger Index: Food Systems Transformation and Local Governance.* Washington, DC: IFPRI, 2022.

Sachs, Jeffrey D., John McArthur, Guido Schmidt-Traub, Margaret Kruk, Chandrika Bahadur, Michael Faye, and Gordon McCord. "Ending Africa's Poverty Trap." *Brookings Papers on Economic Activity* 1 (2004): 117–240.

Sahn, David E., ed. *The Fight against Hunger and Malnutrition: The Role of Food, Agriculture, and Targeted Policies.* New York: Oxford, 2015.

Thurow, Roger. *The Last Hunger Season: A Year in an African Farm Community on the Brink of Change.* New York: Public Affairs, 2012.

US Department of Agriculture. *Household Food Security in the United States 2021.* Economic Research Report ERR-309. Washington, DC: USDA, 2022.

The Politics of Famine

Becker, Jasper. *Hungry Ghosts: Mao's Secret Famine.* New York: Holt, 1998.

Conquest, Robert. *Harvest of Sorrow: Soviet Collectivization and the Terror Famine.* New York: Oxford University Press, 1987.

Grada, Cormac O. *Famine: A Short History.* Princeton, NJ: Princeton University Press, 2009.

Haggard, Stephan, and Marcus Noland. *Famine in North Korea: Markets, Aid, and Reform*. New York: Columbia University Press, 2009.

Natsios, Andrew. *The Great North Korean Famine*. Washington, DC: US Institute of Peace Press, 2002.

Sen, Amartya. *Poverty and Famines: An Essay on Entitlement and Deprivation*. New York: Oxford University Press, 1983.

The Green Revolution Controversy

Altieri, Miguel. *Agroecology: The Science of Sustainable Agriculture*. 2nd ed. Boulder, CO: Westview Press, 1995.

Evenson, R. E., and D. Gollin. "Assessing the Impact of the Green Revolution, 1960 to 2000." *Science* 300 (May 2003): 758–762.

Hayami, Yujiro, and Vernon W. Ruttan. *Agricultural Development: An International Perspective*. Baltimore: Johns Hopkins University Press, 1985.

Hazell, Peter, and Lawrence Haddad. *Agricultural Research and Poverty Reduction*. Food, Agriculture, and Environment Discussion Paper 34. Washington, DC: International Food Policy Research Institute, 2001.

Hazell, Peter, C. Ramasamy, and P. K. Aiyasamy. *The Green Revolution Reconsidered*. Baltimore: Johns Hopkins University Press, 1991.

International Assessment of Agricultural Science, Technology, and Development. *Executive Summary of Synthesis Report*. Washington, DC: Island Press, 2008. http://www.agassessment.org/docs/IAASTD_exec_summary_JAN_2008.pdf.

Juma, Calestous. *The New Harvest: Agricultural Innovation in Africa*. New York: Oxford University Press, 2011.

Pingali, Prabhu L. "Green Revolution: Impacts, Limits, and the Path Ahead." *PNAS* 109, no. 31 (2012): 12302–12308.

Ruttan, Vernon W. "Controversy about Agricultural Technology: Lessons from the Green Revolution." *International Journal of Biotechnology* 6, no. 1 (2004): 43–54.

Williams, Robert G. *Export Agriculture and the Crisis in Central America*. Chapel Hill: University of North Carolina Press, 1986.

Food Aid, Food Power, and Development Assistance

Barrett, Christopher B., Andrea Binder, and Julia Steets, eds. *Uniting on Food Assistance: The Case for Transatlantic Cooperation*. New York: Routledge, 2012.

Barrett, Christopher B., and Daniel G. Maxwell. *Food Aid after Fifty Years: Recasting Its Role*. New York: Routledge, 2005.

Bertini, Catherine, and Dan Glickman. *2012 Progress Report on U.S. Leadership in Global Agricultural Development*. Chicago: Chicago Council on Global Affairs, 2012.

Paarlberg, Robert. *Food Trade and Foreign Policy: India, the Soviet Union, and the United States*. Ithaca, NY: Cornell University Press, 1985.

Riley, Barry. *The Political History of American Food Aid: An Uneasy Benevolence*. New York: Oxford University Press, 2017.

The Politics of Obesity

Fisher, Andrew. *Big Hunger: The Unholy Alliance between Corporate America and Anti-Hunger Groups*. Cambridge, MA: MIT Press, 2018.

Kessler, David A. *The End of Overeating*. Emmaus, PA: Rodale Press, 2009.

Ludwig, David S. "Childhood Obesity—The Shape of Things to Come." *New England Journal of Medicine* 357, no. 23 (2007): 2325–2327.

Moss, Michael. *Hooked: Food, Free Will, and How the Food Giants Exploit Our Addictions*. New York: Random House, 2021.

Nestle, Marion. *Soda Politics: Taking on Big Soda (and Winning)*. New York: Oxford, 2015.

Oliver, J. Eric. *Fat Politics: The Real Story behind America's Obesity Epidemic*. New York: Oxford University Press, 2006.

Popkin, Barry. *The World Is Fat*. New York: Penguin, 2008.

Sassi, Franco. *Obesity and the Economics of Prevention: Fit Not Fat*. Paris: OECD, 2010.

Taubes, Gary. *The Case against Sugar*. New York: Knopf, 2016

The Politics of Farm Subsidies and Trade

Bosso, Christopher. *Framing the Farm Bill: Interests, Ideology, and the Agricultural Act of 2014*. Lawrence: University Press of Kansas, 2017.

Clapp, Jennifer. *Food*. Cambridge, MA: Polity Press, 2012.

Food First. *Food Sovereignty: A Right for All—Political Statement of the NGO/CSO Forum for Food Sovereignty*. Oakland, CA: Food First, 2002.

Gardner, Bruce L. *American Agriculture in the Twentieth Century: How It Flourished and What It Cost*. Cambridge, MA: Harvard University Press, 2002.

Honma, Masayoshi, and Yujiro Hayami. "The Determinants of Agricultural Protection Level: An Econometric Analysis." In *The Political Economy of Agricultural Protection*, edited by Kym Anderson and Yujiro Hayami, 39–49. Sydney: Allen and Unwin, 1986.

Orden, David, Robert Paarlberg, and Terry Roe. *Policy Reform in American Agriculture: Analysis and Prognosis*. Chicago: University of Chicago Press, 1999.

Tracy, Michael. *Government and Agriculture in Western Europe 1880–1988*. 3rd ed. New York: New York University Press, 1989.

Livestock, Meat, and Climate

Ausbel, Jesse H., Iddo K. Wernick, and Paul E. Waggoner. "Peak Farmland and the Prospect for Land Sparing." *Population and Development Review* 38, supplement (2012): 1–28. http://phe.rock efeller.edu/docs/PDR.SUPP%20Final%20Paper.pdf.

Burney, Jennifer, Steven Davis, and David Lobell. "Greenhouse Gas Mitigation by Agricultural Intensification." *PNAS* 107, no. 26 (2010): 12052–12057.

Carson, Rachel. *Silent Spring*. Boston: Houghton Mifflin, 1962.

The EAT-Lancet Commission on Food, Planet, Health. *Summary Report*. Stockholm Resilience Center, Stockholm, 2019. https://eatforum. org/eat-lancet-commission.

Masson, Jeffrey. *The Face on Your Plate: The Truth about Food*. New York: W. W. Norton, 2009.

Nelson, Gerald C., et al. *Climate Change: Impact on Agriculture and Costs of Adaptation*. Washington, DC: IFPRI, 2009.

Norwood, F. Bailey, and Jayson L. Lusk, *Compassion by the Pound: The Economics of Farm Animal Welfare*. New York: Oxford, 2011.

Organisation for Economic Co-operation and Development. *Environmental Performance of Agriculture in OECD Countries since 1990*. Paris: OECD, 2008.

Paarlberg, Robert. *Countrysides at Risk: The Political Geography of Sustainable Agriculture*. Baltimore: Johns Hopkins University Press, 1996.

Pew Trusts. *Sustainable Marine Aquaculture*. Takoma Park, MD: Marine Aquaculture Task Force, 2007.

Shapiro, Paul. *Clean Meat: How Growing Meat without Animals Will Revolutionize Dinner and the World*. New York: Gallery Books, 2018

Waldau, Paul. *Animal Rights: What Everyone Needs to Know*. New York: Oxford University Press, 2011.

Agribusiness, Supermarkets, and Fast Food

Belasco, Warren. *Appetite for Change: How the Counterculture Took on the Food Industry, 1966–1988*. New York: Pantheon, 1989.

Goldberg, Ray A. *Food Citizenship: Food System Advocates in an Era of Distrust*. New York: Oxford University Press, 2018.

Grey, Mark A. "The Industrial Food Stream and Its Alternatives in the United States: An Introduction." *Human Organization* 59, no. 2 (Summer 2000): 143–150.

Reardon, Thomas, C. Peter Timmer, and Julio Berdegue. "The Rapid Rise of Supermarkets in Developing Countries." *Journal of Agricultural and Development Economics* 1, no. 2 (2004): 168–183.

Watson, James. *Golden Arches East: McDonald's in East Asia*. 2nd ed. Stanford, CA: Stanford University Press, 2006.

Organic and Local Food

Counihan, Carole. *Food Culture: A Reader*. 2nd ed. New York: Routledge, 2007.

Fromartz, Samuel. *Organic, Inc*. New York: Harcourt, 2006.

McWilliams, James E. *Just Food*. Boston: Little, Brown, 2009.

Obach, Brian K. *Organic Struggle: The Movement for Sustainable Agriculture in the United States*. Cambridge, MA: MIT Press, 2015

Pollan, Michael. *The Omnivore's Dilemma: A Natural History of Four Meals*. New York: Penguin, 2006.

Ronald, Pamela C., and Raoul W. Adamchak, *Tomorrow's Table: Organic Farming, Genetics, and the Future of Food*. New York: Oxford University Press, 2008.

Smil, Vaclav. "Global Population and the Nitrogen Cycle." *Scientific American* (July 1997): 76–81.

Smil, Vaclav. *Enriching the Earth: Fritz Haber, Carl Bosch, and the Transformation of World Food Production*. Cambridge, MA: MIT Press, 2001.

UNEP-UNCTAD. *Organic Agriculture and Food Security in Africa: Capacity-Building Task Force on Trade, Environment and Development*. New York and Geneva: United Nations, 2008.

USDA. "Local Food Systems: Concepts, Impacts, and Issues." ERS Report 97, May 2010.

Vogt, G. "The Origins of Organic Farming." In *Organic Farming: An International History*, edited by W. Lockeretz, 9–29. Wallingford, UK: CABI, 2008.

Williamson, Claire. "Is Organic Food Better for Our Health?" *Nutrition Bulletin* 32, no. 2 (2007): 104–108.

Winter, Carl K., and Sarah F. Davis. "Organic Foods." *Journal of Food Science* 7, no. 9 (2006): 117–124.

Food Safety and Genetically Engineered Food

Brookes, Graham, and Peter Barfoot. "Environmental Impacts of Genetically Modified (GM) Crop Use 1996–2018: Impacts on Pesticide Use and Carbon Emissions." *GM Crops and Food* 11, no. 4 (2020): 215–241.

Huang, J., R. Hu, C. Fan, C. E. Pray, and S. Rozelle. "*Bt* Cotton Benefits, Costs, and Impacts in China," *AgBioForum* 5, no. 4 (2002): 153–166.

James, Clive. *Global Status of Commercialized Biotech/GM Crops.* ISAAA Brief 39. Ithaca, NY: International Service for the Acquisition of Agribiotech Applications, 2008.

Jasanoff, Sheila. *Designs on Nature: Science and Democracy in Europe and the United States.* Princeton, NJ: Princeton University Press, 2005.

Little, Amanda. *The Fate of Food: What We'll Eat in a Bigger, Hotter, Smarter World.* New York: Harmony, 2019.

Lynas, Mark. *Seeds of Science: Why We Got It So Wrong on GMOs.* London: Bloomsbury Sigma, 2018.

Nestle, Marion. *Safe Food: The Politics of Food Safety.* Berkeley: University of California Press, 2010.

Paarlberg, Robert. *The Politics of Precaution: Genetically Modified Crops in Developing Countries.* Washington, DC: International Food Policy Research Institute, 2001.

Paarlberg, Robert. *Starved for Science: How Biotechnology Is Being Kept Out of Africa.* Cambridge, MA: Harvard University Press, 2008.

Specter, Michael. "Seeds of Doubt: An Activist's Controversial Crusade against Genetically Modified Crops," *New Yorker*, August 18, 2014.

Who Governs the World Food System?

Chicago Council on Global Affairs. *Renewing American Leadership in the Fight against Global Hunger and Poverty.* Chicago: Chicago Council on Global Affairs, 2009.

Duncan, Jessica. *Global Food Security Governance: Civil Society Engagement in the Reformed Committee on World Food Security.* London: Routledge, 2015.

Easterly, William. *The White Man's Burden: Why the West's Efforts to Aid the Rest Have Done So Much Ill and So Little Good.* New York: Penguin, 2007.

IFPRI. *2021 Global Food Policy Report: Transforming Food Systems after COVID-19.* Washington, DC: International Food Policy Research Institute, 2021

IFPRI. *Inclusive Food System Transformations for Healthy Diets: National Experiences with a Global Challenge.* Washington, DC: International Food Policy Research Institute, 2020.

Keck, Margaret E., and Kathryn Sikkink. *Activists beyond Borders: Advocacy Networks in International Politics.* Ithaca, NY: Cornell University Press, 1998.

Paarlberg, Robert. *Governance and Food Security in an Age of Globalization.* Food, Agriculture, and the Environment Discussion Paper 36. Washington, DC: International Food Policy Research Institute, 2002.

INDEX

For the benefit of digital users, indexed terms that span two pages (e.g., 52–53) may, on occasion, appear on only one of those pages.